FLOW

Releasing a River of
Healing into Healthcare

Rhonda Hamilton, APRN

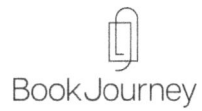

CONTENTS

To my sister Kim Silliker, who first made me a storyteller. When we were children, you'd ask me for a bedtime story every night. Even though you promised to tell me one in return, you usually drifted off to sleep on the pillow beside me before your turn. Those moments shaped me and taught me how to tell a story and how to listen—an ability that has become a part of who I am.

And to my husband, Rick Hamilton, who removed every excuse, every hesitation, and every obstacle right down to the chair I sit in as I write these words. Your unwavering belief in me made me believe in myself.

With love and gratitude, this is for you both.

AUTHOR'S NOTE

God wants to release a river of healing through his Holy Spirit into healthcare. In this book, I share my story and the lessons I've learned in my nearly four decades of nursing—what holds his healing back and what releases it to freely flow. This book is written mostly for those who want to make a difference in healthcare, but it is also written for anyone who has faced health challenges. I invite you to join me in the healing river.

CHAPTER 1
RIVER OF LIFE

I've got a river of life flowing out of me,
Makes the lame to walk and the blind to see,
Opens prison doors sets the captives free.
I've got a river of life flowing out of me.
TRADITIONAL CHRISTIAN SONG[1]

The young pastor had just been diagnosed. His issue was an uncontrolled autoimmune disorder causing severe inflammation, which led to aggressive hepatic cancer. He and his wife came to our weekly meeting for prayer, and now the dejected young man sat slumped on a chair in the middle of the room, tired and defeated.

Here I was, a nurse practitioner currently working in palliative care, facing down a diagnosed case of aggressive cancer. It stared me in the face, reminding me of frail patients I had been caring for. I was dealing with so much death these days. Death can be peaceful, and in some ways quite beautiful, when the patient has lived a full life and is lovingly surrounded by family as they leave pain and suffering behind on earth. At other times, such as death from cancer in a young person with a young family, it is painfully unfair and random. Cancer is such an overpowering disease, it threatens and discourages us from praying, much less with any amount of faith for healing.

My strong inclination for mercy and justice are what led me into nursing. I wanted to minister to the sick, but what did I have to offer my patients besides my medical knowledge, mercy, and empathy? These are beautiful God-given skills that he has given those of us in medicine, yet God had been showing me there is more for us to receive and to offer.

As medical professionals, we are the receivers of the sick. God has positioned us at the frontline, and this presents us with an incredible opportunity to help others on their path to healing. But we are a disappointed group. We have seen so much suffering. We have watched godly people die. We've prayed for the sick and God didn't come through. When we do see or hear about a miraculous healing, we are immediately skeptical, even though deep down in our hearts we really do want to see mighty signs and wonders.

We are Christians who believe the Scriptures and believe Jesus can heal. It's in the Bible. Then why are so many of us afraid or skeptical and faithless in our professional lives as healthcare providers? How did we get here?

There are several reasons, which we will explore together in this book. One of my personal reasons for being doubtful for so much of my life goes all the way back to my childhood.

I come from seven generations of Baptists. Most of my childhood was spent in the province of New Brunswick, Canada, and my church experience as a child was nominal. Our family mostly went to church because it was a part of our culture.

Every summer I filled out the application for Bible camp, and Mom and Dad would scrounge together the hundred dollars it cost to send me and my older sister to Camp Wildwood. They'd drop us off for a week of spiritual immersion to hopefully prop us up for the next school year. I loved Bible camp, and my young soul thrived in the spiritual atmosphere. Camp Wildwood left its mark on me and spoiled me for the real world, because Bible camp world and the real world were two very different places on earth.

Bible camp lived and breathed life. I woke every morning with joy. I felt spiritually renewed and protected from all the harsh elements that I faced in my daily life. As the week ended, I longed to stay there. At Bible camp, we sang the song "I've Got a River of Life" with incredible joy accompanied by comical, dramatized actions. I felt free, uninhibited, and without fear in the presence of complete acceptance and love.

On Saturday, the last day of camp, Mom and Dad would arrive to find me waiting with my rolled-up sleeping bag and suitcase, my Bible clutched to my chest, my crafts and Bible study notes squirreled away in a small bag. I didn't want to leave because I knew what awaited me the next day.

I would go to my traditional Baptist church and sit with my family and sing traditional hymns with an occasional chorus thrown in. I was such a perceptive child and an expert authenticity analyst. I'd watch as the pastor tried to rouse the congregation into the same chorus, "I've Got a River of Life," during the morning service, and look around at mechanical, obedient voices coming from mouths with forced smiles doing uncomfortable robotic, controlled actions to the words of the song. It was never the same as summer camp. Clearly not all Baptist churches are the same, but I didn't experience the life-giving flow of God at ours. Even though we sang about a river of life, it didn't ever seem to flow through our church on Sunday mornings.

The experience I felt at summer camp eventually waned and flickered out after a few weeks at home. Home, school, and church life felt lonely and confusing. During my teen years I rebelled, then turned my life fully over to Jesus at age twenty-two, but I still dealt with anxiety and depression for several years. After high school graduation I went to nursing school, and one year after becoming an RN I got married. My husband, Rick, and I moved to western Canada for work and quickly joined an independent Baptist church.

At first, we gravitated to the church for its commonality, falling comfortably into submission to familiar Christian cultural norms. We followed the established church standards without question. We sang about the "River of Life" but we didn't know what it really meant.

Years later, all of this would change. After I had been married and working as a nurse for several years, God began to prompt Rick and me to ask questions. Most of them revolved around this: Why is it that the beliefs and actions we see at church aren't matching what we read in the Bible? At the time, we didn't know that our journey to experiencing the true River of Life had begun. Over the next several years, I learned that the Holy Spirit *is* the River of Life, and that he is present and active in our lives.

ENGAGING WITH THE FLOW

We called my great-grandmother "Gramma." I didn't know her real name, but I remember her as a stout, old woman with long, gray hair that she wore pinned up on her head like a loose crown. She lived on a hill in eastern Canada without electricity or running water until she died in the 1970s. It is a special place we still call "The Hill."

After summer camp our family would get together on The Hill with other available family members and help my grandfather bring in the hay for the winter. My job as a child was to stomp and pack the loose hay into the hay wagon until it was so high I felt like I was sitting on a rough, scratchy, wobbly cloud. Grampy would pull us with the tractor from The Hill to his own barn in the village a few miles away. I sat on the pinnacle of the swaying heap waving to the neighbors like a conqueror of the harvest.

The best memory of those hot, sweaty haymaking days centers around the rusty, brown metal hand pump up on The Hill. The water from the well was unlike the water we drank at home; it was cold, fresh, and thirst quenching, and it was even better when we drank it from the blue metallic aluminum cup that Nanny said she bought from a traveling salesman. The pump required some hard, fast pumping. I remember jumping into the air and using the weight of my small body to maximize my efforts on the pump handle until a satisfying stream of water burst forth from the spout. If my sister was there, she'd keep pumping so I could put my whole head under the pump for a few seconds to cool off before the cold water made my head begin to ache.

If the pump hadn't been used for a while, it needed to be primed. Priming is all about getting rid of air in the pump to create the necessary suction required to draw water. When the pump needed to be primed, I'd grab some rainwater from a nearby water barrel and pour it down the top of the handpump while pumping furiously until I felt the pump start to draw—a sensation that is better felt than "telt," as Grampy would say. Until the pump is primed, the handle feels light and weightless and pumping is easy, just without getting any water. Once the water engages, the pull on the pump handle becomes weighty and heavier, requiring greater strength to pull the handle. Sometimes I needed to go back to the water barrel a few times before I was successful in getting the pump to prime, but eventually I could feel the catch, or the weight of the draw. The draw became smoother, longer, and intentional, and I could feel the water coming up from the depths of the well.

There is a high sense of anticipation that follows the weight on the handle, and it filled me with a renewed sense of purpose and energy. A person could pump all day, but if they don't ever experience the weighty drawing sensation on the water pump handle, they won't get a drop of water. The barrier of air prevents the water from being able to flow freely.

It has taken a lifetime for me to know and understand the empty spiritual feeling of a dry pump compared to the weighty sensation of the approaching flow of the Holy Spirit. At times I haven't primed the spiritual pump enough, allowing the barrier of old fear, skepticism, or doubt to prevent the draw. But I'm learning how to keep pressing in. I can't make it happen on my own; however, it seems like my willingness, awareness, and readiness serve to help prime the pump and are directly related to the flow of the Holy Spirit from within me. Every time I feel the weight of the draw of the Holy Spirit, I am reminded that miracles are "not by might, nor by power, but by my Spirit" (Zechariah 4:6).

Now, back to the young pastor recently diagnosed with cancer. At our prayer meeting, we prayed fervently for him. I bounced between shame for my skepticism and fear that we were offering false hope to a cancer patient. How could I be so unbelieving? Stepping onto a precipice of faith could hurt me in the end. It had hurt me so many times before.

Memories of disappointment, mixed with a restrictive, deep-rooted theology from my upbringing, threatened to sabotage my newfound faith. My medical knowledge fueled the doubts; I knew that if left untreated, hepatocellular carcinoma was very aggressive.

It was easier for me to shrink back into a "will of God" stance, a coping mechanism many of us lean on when dealing with sick patients. When all else fails, we pray for the will of God, or we pray for patience and comfort so that everyone feels good about the visit. We feel good because we did something spiritual, and the patient feels reassured and loved. The "will of God" prayer is much safer in situations like this. It's safer for me, protecting me from disappointment, and for my patients and their loved ones, not giving false hope.

One of my patients who was struggling with a difficult diagnosis was called forward in a church service so the congregation could lay hands on him and pray for healing. Each person who prayed said the same thing: "God, if it be your will, please heal this man!" He told me he sat there thinking, *These are not prayers for healing. They are not asking God for anything!*

Are these prayers a partnership with God, or are they safe prayers that come from our own sense of helplessness? There is no chance of failure when we push all the responsibility back on God.

What is the prayer of faith spoken of in James 5:15–16? James says, "Is any sick among you? let him call for the elders of the church; and let them pray over him, anointing him with oil in the name of the Lord: and the prayer of faith shall save the sick, and the Lord shall raise him up; and if he has committed sins, they shall be forgiven him" (KJV).

The prayer of faith is characterized by trust and confidence in God's ability to bring about the very thing we ask for. Faith is work. The prayer of faith requires a work of faith, much like the diligent effort of going to the source of water to prime the pump. It's easier to slip into a "will of God" prayer that doesn't leave us disappointed or get people's hopes up. But while it's safer, it is also not very effective. We can pump and pray, but without priming and opening the way for the Holy Spirit, nothing will flow.

Over the few months after the young pastor's cancer diagnosis, I had begun to experience the flow of the Holy Spirit, and I wanted that same healing experience for this pastor. As part of priming the spiritual pump in prayer, I had to ask myself the tough questions: Do I believe God is good? Do I believe he wants to alleviate suffering and heal the sick? The only hope for this pastor was the healing river that can only come from God himself.

I stepped out in faith in my own prayers, taking risky steps that never would have happened in my early years of nursing, but steps that now placed trust in God's river of healing through the Holy Spirit. This was my first experience of prayer that led to a clinically documented healing. If it were not for the support, freedom, and safety I felt in this small prayer group, I'm not sure I would have learned the ways in which the Holy Spirit spoke to me. The Holy Spirit speaks to us in a way that is personal to us, and has meaning and makes sense to us but may seem odd or unusual to others. Being in a safe mentorship with experienced prayer warriors can allow us to take risks and step out by faith into what God is saying to us or asking us to do.

As I faced the young pastor, the cancer seemed to scream at me, "It's a done deal!" I gave myself a quick pep talk. "Okay, this is not about me coming up with some sort of plan. It is listening and seeing and acting on what the Holy Spirit speaks."

Beside me stood a nursing student, Joel. He was unusual in the ways he heard the Holy Spirit. Sometimes I laughed out loud as he spoke out prayers and prophecy, but I learned to admire him for his courage, sincerity, and accuracy in revealing what was in the hearts of those he prayed for. We stood together—two healthcare professionals in front of a case that seemed hopeless—not with doctors' notes or medical equipment but in Holy Spirit–inspired prayer.

At one point as we were praying, I felt led to turn a golden key on and off inside what appeared to be a flashing oval labyrinth inside the pastor's chest. As I stood in front of the pastor, I turned an invisible-to-the-eye key against his chest. Even as I acted in obedience to what I was sensing, my logical, scientific brain asked, *Are you out of your freaking mind?* Despite my limited faith, I pushed through the protests of my brain and performed the most illogical action I've ever done as a medical professional.

Then Joel, who never failed to surprise me, said he saw some scattered diamond mushrooms left behind. He described them in what, to me, was comical detail. *Are you kidding me?* my brain asked. He felt led to prayerfully remove them. Eyes wide, I stared at the student as if what he said was even crazier than what I had just done. Then I looked at all the solemn, earnest faces in our circle. No one was laughing.

Joel asked the young pastor, "Is it okay if I pull these out? They look valuable, but that's only a trick to make you want to keep them."

Now totally engaged in this exercise, the pastor blurted out, "Yes! Please! Pull them out."

With a kind smile, Joel reached down where the pastor was sitting and performed the action of pulling out the glittering items from the young man's chest. "There. It's done."

We wrapped up our prayer time and each of us headed home. I did so in a daze. This whole thing was crazy, and my mind was trying to make sense of what I had experienced. Honestly, I was fighting incredulous shock and skepticism. The whole experience was comical and bizarre, and I questioned my own sanity.

I couldn't seem to get the image of the flashing labyrinth out of my mind. It was still there in my head, the oval shape with its swollen abdomen moving and flashing like a nighttime view of a bustling metropolis. I had seen this before. It was familiar but I couldn't seem to place it. Again, a vision came into my imagination. A biology textbook fell open to a chapter on the human cell.

There it was. The flashing oval blob. The one I turned off with a golden key. It was a diagram of the human cell, its rough endoplasmic reticulum and Golgi apparatus filling its center like rows of a labyrinth. I could never remember these things in biology class. God had to bring the textbook to me and tell me what had transpired.

I sensed God telling me, "Rhonda, you rebooted him at the cellular level. That is what I asked you to do. Joel picked out all the remaining cancer cells that were left after the reboot." It all made perfect sense! I called our group leader the next day to tell him what I had seen. I learned that God doesn't always speak to us in expected ways—the way we think God *should* speak to us. This was my very first experience in allowing myself to see the unusual way the Holy Spirit communicated, and my first time following his lead the way my mentors were. I trusted I was doing the right thing, and it turns out I did exactly what God showed me.

We didn't hear from the young pastor for about three or four months. He finally came back to follow up with a report on his health condition. He informed us his spiral into cancer treatment came to a halt. When he followed up with tests, his gastroenterologist said to him, "I don't know what happened, but it's like you've been rebooted at the cellular level." There was no cancer, no inflammation.

The young pastor wanted to push things further with the specialist. He asked, "Does that mean I can start eating bread again?"

The flustered specialist stammered, "Well, let's not push things too far!"

The results of this prophetic act that led to healing hit me like an open fire hydrant. I wanted to believe, but I sat there stunned. The clinical results of the imaging, the comment of the specialist, and the loud echo of hallelujahs emerging from our small group who had prayed could not drown out my doubts and skepticism when it came to believing this young pastor was healed. Would it last? Was it real?

Echoes from years of disappointment, strict doctrine, and compiled medical knowledge still made me doubt. But I could not deny what had taken place. The steps toward eradicating the cancer in this young pastor's body extended beyond anything I'd learned in school or in medical practice. I could choose to ignore what I'd seen, or I could embrace the undeniable interaction with the Holy Spirit that resulted in a miraculous healing—the kind of healings Jesus performed in the Bible and promises for us today.

I saw the problem now. If I couldn't push forward with my spiritual gifts in my medical profession, then all I could offer my patients was a practice largely based on medical research without the wisdom, comfort, and healing power that flows from the Holy Spirit living within us. God wants to open a river of healing that flows into health-care, and he wants it to flow through us.

Jesus offers to release a river of healing through the Holy Spirit into the dry places of disappointment and skepticism that not only exist in the healthcare field, but also in the lives of anyone who has encountered health challenges. In the book of John, we see how Jesus cried out to the crowd:

"If anyone thirsts, let him come to Me and drink. He who believes in Me, as the Scripture has said, out of his heart will flow rivers of living water." But this He spoke concerning the Spirit, whom those believing in Him would receive. (John 7:37–39 NKJV)

Although I was new at experiencing the healing flow in such an unusual way—with flashing blobs and diamond mushrooms—the Spirit worked through me that evening, and he has continued to lead me in similar prayers.

I was mentored by a group of people who had been utilizing their gifts of prophecy and healing together for seventeen years, and they provided a safe place for me to take risks, to gently walk out my own gifts that had been suppressed or not activated for years because of my theology. At times I thought it was over the top (seriously, diamond mushrooms?), but I saw the results of these prayer times. People walked out of the room healed, edified, and loved.

It broke my rigidity and group conformity to be able to hear God in the way he spoke to me personally. While praying with my mentors I heard words spoken over people that God himself could only know, and I saw people break down in tears feeling completely seen and heard by God. These times were incredibly beautiful. The prophecy was done in love. Because of this group helping me accept the flow of the Holy Spirit through me, I have been able to step out by faith and do the same.

That Monday night of prayer over a discouraged cancer patient primed the pump for living water more than any of us knew. Shortly after this health crisis, the young pastor moved with his wife and family to a new ministry. I have followed his life on Instagram because, to be honest, I want to ensure he is still healthy. As healthcare professionals we tend to want to know if the healing "stuck." I recently supported him this past year as he traveled to Mexico again to work with YWAM (Youth With A Mission) and build homes for the poor.

Since that first clinically diagnosed healing, I've grown in my faith when it comes to collaborating with the Holy Spirit in my family practice. There is a river of healing. Many of us think this river is some mystical, magical place in a land far away guarded by angels with flaming swords of fire. No. This far-off, obscure river is much closer than we can understand or comprehend. The river is within us.

CHAPTER 2

DISAPPOINTMENTS AND DRUGS

I find your lack of faith disturbing.

DARTH VADER, *STAR WARS EPISODE IV: A NEW HOPE*

R ather than focusing on our skepticisms and doubts, it's better to identify possible reasons for our struggle with faith. Why do we resist releasing the Holy Spirit within our professional vocations? Two of the main reasons why those of us in healthcare struggle to believe Jesus can use us to bring healing to the sick are disappointment and our perspective of medical science. I've had to recognize and deal with both of these in my own life.

DISAPPOINTMENT

We were young. We were newly married. And we were financially broke. I had graduated as an RN a year before Rick and I married, then after marriage we quickly started having babies. Two years in, Rick suffered a neck injury that required surgery and several months out of work. He was unemployed and I was home with two children. We could barely pay the rent. Kind people who knew our situation occasionally dropped food donations on our doorstep.

We lived in Canada at the time, and both Rick and I were hunters. With a steady supply of deer meat frozen, and since large bags of rice were cheap, our meal plan rarely changed. Rick's mother had lived through the depression and tended to buy sale items and then freeze them for possible future destitution. As a widow who didn't require much food, her freezer became a time capsule of odd and unusual sale items, and we became the beneficiaries. Several weeks of deer meat and rice combined with odd frozen vegetable sides became a test of contentment, and we both found ourselves somewhat empathetic with the relationship the children of Israel had with manna.

After weeks of dietary monotony, an invitation for dinner with friends came as a relief. We piled into the vehicle, excited to escape deer meat and rice with a side dish from the antiquated freezer. When we arrived, our friends excitedly shared the menu for this evening's meal. Someone had given them some deer meat, and they were so excited to share the delicacy with us on a bed of rice. Rick and I could only stare at each other across the table while feigning gratefulness and complimenting the cook on the great delicious meal.

Back home, our murmuring eventually came to a crescendo. The final straw came sometime later, associated with the last of the odd freezer bags donated by Rick's mother. It was a ball of frozen, freezer-dried cauliflower. I tried my best but couldn't rid it of its pale, whitish-gray appearance or its tasteless, dry, chewy texture. I looked across the dinner table at Rick chewing silently. "I don't know what I'm eating," he muttered, and I started to cry. Shortly after that intolerable meal, Rick announced, "We are going out for dinner!" He wanted to take me to one of the most expensive restaurants in our city, and he was confident God would give us the money to pay for it. I wanted to believe. And I felt ashamed of my fearfulness.

"We're going out for dinner and we're going to trust God to provide!" Rick couldn't help himself. He was rescuing his new wife from despondency, two babies, and a dwindling food supply.

After we dropped off our babies with some friends, we walked into the restaurant dressed in our finest. No one would ever have guessed that our wallets were empty. With great bravado, Rick checked in under our reservation and we were led to a quiet, romantic table for two. I could feel my heart racing. The menu was shaking slightly while I stared at the prices of the entrées.

We ordered a fine dinner and Rick appeared so confident. He kept repeating, "God will provide," but I wasn't tasting the food. I was trying desperately to steady my hand so my food would stay on my fork before it made it into my mouth. I kept looking around the restaurant for God's provision. Whenever someone walked by our table, I would look to see whether they were going to drop money in front of us. I even looked under the table for money.

After we finished eating, we sat for another thirty minutes waiting in silence for God to provide. Finally, Rick stood and we walked toward the exit in silence. He told the server that he'd forgotten his wallet, and I sat down on a bench as collateral under the watchful eye of the cashier. I was embarrassed, humiliated, and feeling so stupid for believing something that didn't materialize. God did not come through. God did not provide, and the miracle did not happen.

Rick sheepishly walked back into the restaurant about fifteen minutes later with a credit card, paid for the meal, and redeemed me from the server's bench.

As soon as we were out the door, I turned to him. "Whose credit card do you have?"

He self-consciously answered, "My friend Daryl happened to be working at the Dairy Queen next door. I told him what happened, and he let me borrow his credit card. We need to pay him back later."

Still not the miracle we had hoped for, but at least we saved face from public humiliation, and I don't think Daryl was aware of our blunder. This story occurred almost forty years ago, and yes, we did pay back Daryl when we finally were able to get some money together.

Both Rick and I laugh about this story and have forgiven our youthful selves. Acts of faith that end in disappointment are our coming-of-age stories in our walk of faith.

It took some time for me to trust my husband again. It has taken a lifetime for me to trust God, but this life journey is a series of choices to believe. I could have stopped at the beginning, never believing in my husband ever again. I could have held this situation against him, critical of his leadership, challenging his direction from God, but I would never have the marriage I have today. I could have walked away from God because, for whatever reason, he did not provide like we thought he would, but I would never have the faith journey that I experience today.

What does this mean for those of us called into healthcare to minister to the sick?

Do we want to see people healed? Yes, we do! We long for it. We are like little children standing in front of the candy store window. The candy is inside. We want the candy, but we don't bother checking our pockets because the last time we reached in they were empty. We step out in faith, believing God will certainly heal our patient just like two newlyweds who bank on him paying for their much-needed meal, only to be stuck with the tab of disappointment. We've witnessed patients with great faith succumb to terminal diagnoses. With discouragement, we've seen faith-filled prayers appear to go unanswered. We watch as heartbeats slow and organs shut down, helpless to do anything to stop any of it. Yes, as healthcare workers we have good reason to be skeptical.

Do we still believe God provides, despite the multitude of disappointments breathing down our neck that remind us of the pain and humiliation associated with broken dreams?

When we start down this road of faith, we will encounter several forks. There is always one road that is wider and well-traveled and wisely named Disappointment Street. It leads to Bitterness Avenue and the Twin Cities of Skepticism and Pessimism.

The other path seems narrower and has more overgrowth. Tall grass is springing up between the ruts in the pathway, and wisps of flimsy branches whip across my face. This worn, narrow path is called Faith Way. There are little rest stops along the way called Places of Grace. The road eventually gets wider and more clearly marked, but there are still opportunities to take the next exit to catch Disappointment Street. Confronting the sick and suffering is a series of forks stuck in our walk of faith. We choose every day where we will put our trust.

Today, Rick and I live in Kona, Hawaii. Our five children (we had five in five years!) are grown and no longer under our roof. Rick works with YWAM, and I am the medical director of a nonprofit health organization. We've come a long way from our deer and rice and mystery frozen veggie days. There have been many forks in the road for us—and lots of disappointment, yes—but also much joy and many spiritual lessons flowing along the way.

When we let past disappointments guide our thoughts and beliefs about healing, it is like pumping an unprimed pump. Disappointment becomes the air blocking the flow of the Holy Spirit from engaging. If we continue to expect to be disappointed, we most likely will be.

OUR PERSPECTIVE ON MEDICAL SCIENCE

The struggle with skepticism and lack of faith in the medical field is real. I once sat beside an elderly gentleman at a prophetic conference. When I confided in him about my struggle with faith, he looked at me with surprise. "Your medical background is messing you up!" he told me.

I pondered his blunt answer and lack of empathy during my vulnerable confession. Maybe he was right. Perhaps I wouldn't struggle with a lack of faith if I wasn't educated in science and medicine. It could be that my medical knowledge and experience reduce my faith in God's healing power. Maybe a prayer of faith for healing would be easier if I hadn't encountered so much sickness and suffering as a healthcare professional. Perhaps ignorance is bliss. Despite my faith struggles, God has uniquely positioned me as a receiver of the sick. I have a license that gives me medical authority and places me in a position of trust with all my clients. A skilled medical background is essential for my job.

Still, for educated healthcare professionals, our perspective of medical science can create resistance to the healing flow of the Holy Spirit. Trusting the scientific process, we immediately go into medical mode and diagnose the illness, order all the necessary labs, and prescribe the correct medicine. Don't get me wrong; I love science. I love evidence-based medicine. Reading research articles can be like detective work for my inquisitive mind. I can easily get lost in research, and it can be a deep hole of distraction and hyperfocus for me. My husband has found me sitting on the bed surrounded by piles of studies peppered with sticky notes and marked up with so much high-lighter that it's difficult to know what exactly stood out on the paper.

I recently purchased a lengthy medical resource. The day it arrived in the mail, I opened the package with delight and rubbed my hands over its glossy cover. The pages are busy, the font is small, there are diagrams—and *goodness*, there are algorithms! I can get lost in these pages for hours. The book is lovely and thick, and pages are turned on a large coil spring, with lists of every available medication we use in healthcare. It includes every research article associated with each one so I can decide whether there is good evidence and research that supports the medication I'm considering. My nurse practitioner heart hungers after solutions for the sick. I study research constantly. I believe in the science of medicine.

I also believe that every good gift, such as scientific advances, comes from the Great Healer himself. Some people take this truth to the extreme, believing that since God is Healer, they will accept no other form of treatment. They are suspicious of medicine and place the focus on Jesus only for supernatural healing. Of course, they will also accept natural supplements and herbs or alternative forms of healing since these were created by God and are acceptable and therefore more spiritual.

Throughout the Word of God are verses that tell us about herbs and nutrition that bring healing, speaking of the natural healing that is available in our God-given bodies, as well as the power of a positive outlook and cheerful heart (see Ezekiel 47:12; Psalm 104:15). The psalmist wrote,

> He waters the hills from His upper chambers; the earth is satis-
> fied with the fruit of Your works. He causes the grass to grow

for the cattle, and vegetation for the service of man, that he may bring forth food from the earth, and wine that makes glad the heart of man, oil to make his face shine, and bread which strengthens man's heart. (Psalm 104:13–15 NKJV)

There are individuals whom I admire on Instagram and YouTube who have devoted their lives to the study of alternative medicine. I know there are untapped treasures found in herbs and nutrition that are often underrated, especially in our Western world. Remedies that have been passed down through generations have valid healing properties. I admit I lack wisdom and experience in this area of alternative medicine, but I value its role in healing.

I have also seen its successes. A recent patient of mine had a terrible fungal infection in his finger- and toenails. Over the counter creams and remedies did not resolve his problem, and expensive prescriptions did not work either. He finally went to a naturopath who told him his fungal infection was in his body. They recommended hyperbaric oxygen therapy at their clinic. It would take months and the cost would be exorbitant. Months later, this patient returned to my clinic with clear, beautiful nails. He explained he couldn't afford to pay for the hyperbaric treatments, so he researched the cost of purchasing a hyperbaric chamber for himself. He was retired, so he got a part-time job at a large retail store in town and saved his paychecks until he had enough money to purchase the $8,000 machine online. He set it up in his spare bedroom and gave himself treatments just as the naturopath clinic had recommended. I looked at his nails and shook my head with wonder.

Healing is incredibly complex. Our education, experiences, personal bias, and religious practices can influence where we run to in the face of difficult or desperate diagnoses. While the science of medicine faces its alternative medicine opponent with suspicion, their followers engage in accusatory mudslinging theories of snake oil versus Big Pharma. Although these paradigms can face each other with suspicion, I am convinced there is good wisdom in each that is God-given.

I admit I can quickly run to medical science and pharmaceuticals for answers. Others may run to alternative medicine and remedies that align with their preference for natural healing. However, both conventional and alternative medicines have their strengths and limitations. Integrating elements from either or both paradigms can benefit healing.

GOOD INNER MEDICINE

What about the power of a healthy mind? King Solomon says, "A joyful heart is a good medicine, but a crushed spirit dries up the bones" (Proverbs 17:22). He repeats a similar message in Proverbs 14:30: "A heart at peace gives life to the body, but envy rots the bones" (NIV). Mental health is likely the most important component of healing.

Prescriptions for gratefulness, thankfulness, forgiveness, peace, and love are medicines available for free at the "Working On Myself Pharmacy," the "Making Myself Take Part in Inner Healing Pharmacy," or the "I Will Stop Running from My Trauma Pharmacy." Reflective exploration into our past takes work, and if we are getting professional therapy, it means we must become vulnerable with someone else. There may be a cultural or a generational age group norm that feels stoicism or privacy is more important than exposing that part of ourselves to someone else. Maybe we were raised to keep family secrets to ourselves, and exposure of these things would feel like disloyalty to those we swore to protect. But mental health wounds can be like a sliver causing an infection or a cavity causing a toothache.

Sometimes it takes a professional to objectively pry out the roots of injury to our mental health. Therapists use skilled training to dig out foreign objects or diseased and broken areas in our mind. This type of inner work is not easy. Often, we have to deal with issues we have suppressed throughout our lives. Inner healing can take time, something we don't like to spend on our mental health. However, whether with a qualified counselor or on our own, seeking out past hurts and embedded thoughts is often necessary to have a healthy mind.

For most of my life I have dealt with anxiety. While I was attending

Discipleship Training School at YWAM in 2016, I discovered the guilty root as a buried memory resurfaced.

I was nine years old and standing on the corner of a busy intersection beside a barbershop. I remember that day well. While Dad paid for the haircut, my sweet four-year-old brother walked out of the barbershop to stand beside me. This cute, pudgy little boy behaved so well while getting his haircut that the barber had given him two suckers for sitting still. My brother's chubby hand proudly displayed his reward.

I asked him nicely, "Can you give me one?"

"No! They're mine!" he shouted.

I lunged forward to grab a sucker out of his hand, but he ran—directly into the street and into the path of a car. I heard the ring of the cash register as my dad paid for the haircut. I heard the screech of the tires as the driver hit the brakes. I heard the dull thud of the car hitting my little brother. I saw his limp body catapulted into the air and then land and roll like a lifeless ragdoll in the busy intersection.

Then all was silent. All the cars had stopped. It seemed like time stood still. Traffic was shocked into stillness. It was then that I heard the agonizing scream of my father as he ran from the small barbershop into the intersection to cradle my brother's bloody body.

As I watched this movie in my mind during Discipleship Training School, I saw my nine-year-old self standing silently on the sidewalk watching this traumatic event with expressionless shock. Then I saw a hand from heaven come down and point at my nine-year-old chest, and I heard God quietly say to me, "Rhonda, this is where you were bent."

God was showing me that I was not broken when I was born. I was bent by a traumatic childhood event that left me with a need for perfectionism and for the approval of others. I messed up, not only failing to protect my little brother but sending him into harm's way. My little nine-year-old brain set me on a course of perfectionism, of seeking to please people and to not fail anyone ever again.

It's impossible to avoid failure, so when I did fail people I would run. Run from situations, run from relationships, and run from community. This was the root cause of my anxiety and depression, and it took forty-five years to discover that I didn't know what I didn't know.

Our family experienced a miracle that day so many years ago. While my brother lay in a hospital bed in intensive care, my father went for a walk by himself, crying out to God in desperation. He told us later that it was the one time in his life when he heard the audible voice of God speak from heaven. He heard God say two words: "He'll live." And my brother did. The miracle of this horrific accident was that the only damage to his small body was a severely broken nose that required some reconstructive surgery as he grew older. Today, my brother, Wade, lives back on The Hill with our elderly mother so she is not alone in the family home.

Once we discover complex root causes of illness and emotional pain, God can help us with the rest if we are willing to work on it. I walked through personal forgiveness and experienced a personality change. The anxiety left and I've never been the same. I have had episodes or short seasons where it has tried to return, but when I'm able to identify it and remember that this is not who I am, I'm able to return to a place of peace.

———

As healthcare professionals, we can spend an entire lifetime running after medical science or alternative natural remedies, or learning all we can about inner healing therapies, but healing ultimately comes from God. Regardless of one's belief about medicine, none of us will see the abundant fruit that comes from a partnership with the Holy Spirit unless we open our hearts and minds to receiving his river of healing and allow it to flow through us.

CHAPTER 3
TROUBLE WITH THEOLOGY

Don't wrestle, just nestle.
CORRIE TEN BOOM

W hy is he breathing like this?!" The woman's voice hinged on hysteria.

I stared at her husband thrashing wildly in the hospital bed, a shell of a man who hinted former distinction, writhing frantically like a captured animal. While my patient tore violently at his IV and oxygen tubing, gasping for breath, terrified, I computed signs and symptoms: gulping, clenching, respirations over 60 per minute. His previous nurses told me they had never seen such a low hemoglobin—one of those rare low lab results that you mark down in the Lab Result Hall of Fame. *The lowest hemoglobin ever!* Bragged about in future nursing stories: "I remember when we had a patient with hemoglobin of 20 . . ."

I chose my answer carefully, knowing the patient and his wife were of a religious denomination that refused blood transfusions. "It's because his red blood cell count is so low. These blood cells carry oxygen in the body, and because it's so low the body compensates by increasing respirations."

I caught her grimace of irritation. "Well, can't you do something for him to calm him down?" She tried to compose herself. "I mean, I just can't continue to hold him in the bed like this!" She was frightened and on the verge of tears.

The patient's desperation and struggle for breath made me feel nauseous. I'd been informed that earlier efforts with sedatives had failed to calm him, yet I welcomed the opportunity to leave the room, so I made a dash for the doctor on call to beg for a stronger drug. When I returned with an injection, the wife was still wrestling with her husband. I quickly administered the drug, but even the most powerful medication could not calm this patient who, like a drowning man, fought for life.

For two hours I sat there, a helpless spectator watching a man whose religious convictions allowed the very life to be sucked out of his body. I knew a unit of life-giving blood would see his skin grow pink and his respirations become slow and easy. Instead, his breaths came in gasps, the effort futile, and he simply stopped struggling.

His wife looked at me in a sort of trance and robotically muttered, "He's dying now, isn't he?"

I struggled to answer her. "I think so."

The whole process was horrific to watch. Respirations that were once 50 now came in short grunts every fifteen seconds. His slowing rhythmic respirations resembled the bent wheel on a crashed bicycle, continuing to spin but making a dull sound every time the wheel hit the fender.

The room grew silent except for the buzz of the IV pump and the rush of oxygen through the tubing.

"Is he gone?" she whispered.

"I . . . I . . . think . . . so," I stammered.

She threw herself onto his chest, sobbing uncontrollably. At that moment his motionless body took one last huge gasp of breath, causing the wife to scream and sending my heart into my throat. Momentary terror replaced classic mourning. We stood in shock as he released his last breath, a forever breath, an endless exhale that culminated in a rattling sound.

I walked around the room in a daze, disconnecting tubes and shutting off noisy machines. Gently, I put my hand on her shoulders that shook with grief. "I'm so sorry."

She gave no answer, just quiet sobs. I stood there for a few moments and then left her alone to grieve.

The whole thing was too much for me. I numbly walked to the nurses' station in a fog. What had happened? I tried to cry, to feel upset. What was I feeling? I was empty of all emotion and knew I couldn't go back into that room and offer any sympathy. That was when the tears came, tears because of my inability to offer comfort. "Oh God . . . Oh God . . . I find this so hard."

The memories of that night haunted me for three days. I couldn't seem to push the horrific images from my mind—the bent bicycle tire spinning, scraping the fender; the gasps; the futility. I thought about the religious conviction that refused life-giving blood, resulting in the death of a man's body. Even though I took pride in being impartial in my nursing care, I was still seething with judgment and frustration toward this family over a loss that seemed preventable.

God seemed silent, letting me stew, leaving me to meditate. Were there any winners in this story? Was there any difference between the patient who refused a medical treatment and the young, burned-out nurse trying to bring healing and comfort to patients without the life-giving power of his Spirit?

The lesson came ever so quietly. Everything has a message if we hear it. Both tragedy and beauty speak to those who choose to listen, even if we don't catch the meaning in the moment. Eventually the meaning, the illustration, came softly, quietly, with marvel that his voice came so sweetly, so empathetically. God described to me that he understood my sense of helplessness—because he stands helplessly watching our religious convictions suck spiritual life from our souls.

How horrific for God to watch us refuse his life, refuse the power of his blood that gives strength and power. What desperation he feels when we compensate with an increase in activity, service, and ministry that in the end results in spiritual and physical exhaustion. Meanwhile,

God sits and waits to hang the blood that brings healing and abundant life.

My heart bowed in surrender. I know what it feels like to cling to beliefs so tightly that we lose connection to the source of life.

I appreciate my Baptist roots, specifically the heavy emphasis on the study of the Word of God, but I believe some of my Baptist theology was reactionary to the Pentecostal or charismatic movements. One of the damaging teachings that affected my view and under-standing of the Holy Spirit was taken from this verse:

> Howbeit when he, the Spirit of truth, is come, he will guide you into all truth: for he shall not speak of himself; but whatsoever he shall hear, that he shall speak; and he will shew you things to come. (John 16:13 KJV)

I was taught to be very careful about overemphasizing the Holy Spirit. After all, he doesn't even talk about himself, and he always glorifies Jesus. In other words, you could go wrong by worshipping the Holy Spirit too much. It may make you too emotional, where you become fixated and hung up on the gifts that he has given each of us rather than focusing on Jesus. Even though I was taught that the Holy Spirit is God, this caution inadvertently kept me from experiencing the fullness of the Spirit, because I kept him at careful arm's length out of a sincere desire to please Jesus.

This type of teaching insidiously infers that an overfocus on the Holy Spirit may lead you astray, when Jesus clearly tells us he (Holy Spirit) guides us into the truth (see John 16:13). Placing fear or caution around the Holy Spirit makes him appear untrustworthy. Did I think Jesus or his Father would get jealous and smite me if I focused too much on the Holy Spirit? This type of teaching not only creates fear but reduces the Holy Spirit into a fuel-like mist that performs a secondary function of God instead of being God himself living in us. Besides that, the Holy Spirit doesn't want us to worship him; he wants us to worship Jesus.

The entire chapter of John 16 is about the interdependency

between the Father, Son, and Holy Spirit, and Jesus often referred to himself as the Holy Spirit; he frequently interchanged the use of pronouns. He told the disciples he had to go away so that the Holy Spirit could come. He also assured his disciples he would not leave them alone: "I [Jesus] will not leave you comfortless: I [Holy Spirit] will come to you" (John 14:18 KJV). Jesus was God with us, but the Holy Spirit is God in us. Jesus needed the Holy Spirit; in fact, there is no record in the Bible of any miracles performed by Jesus until after his baptism when he was filled with the Holy Spirit.

> As soon as Jesus was baptized, he went up out of the water. At that moment heaven was opened, and he saw the Spirit of God descending like a dove and alighting upon him. And a voice from heaven said, "This is my Son, whom I love; with him I am well pleased." (Matthew 3:16–17 NIV)

Jesus was full of the Holy Spirit (see Luke 4:1), led of the Holy Spirit (see Matthew 4:1), empowered by the Holy Spirit (see Luke 4:14), and anointed by the Holy Spirit to do ministry (see Luke 4:18–19). Jesus needed the Holy Spirit to fulfill his ministry on earth.

It was the Holy Spirit who led Jesus into the wilderness, who helped him through his forty days of fasting and his temptation. It was the Holy Spirit whom he depended upon on earth to perform all the miracles during his short ministry on earth. Finally, after his death and burial, it was the Holy Spirit who raised Jesus from the dead and took him to heaven, dropped him off, and returned to earth to live in us (see Romans 8:11; John 16:7; Acts 2:1–4). If Jesus needed the Holy Spirit, then how much more do we need him? And doesn't that include the gifts that flow through the Holy Spirit as well?

As a Baptist, I was well versed in the doctrine of cessation. Cessation is the theological belief that certain spiritual gifts, particularly those described in the New Testament, have ceased, or ceased to operate in the same way as they did in the early church, because they were only needed for a specific time. To put it another way, they reached their expiration date. These spiritual gifts can include

speaking in tongues, prophecy, healing, miracles, and more. The belief
is often alluded to from a single passage of Scripture:

> Love never fails. But whether there are prophecies, they will
> fail; whether there are tongues, they will cease; whether there
> is knowledge, it will vanish away. For we know in part and we
> prophesy in part. But when that which is perfect has come, then
> that which is in part will be done away. (1 Corinthians 13:8–10
> NKJV).

Some theologians believe these verses suggest that certain spiritual
gifts would *cease* when *the perfect*, or the completion of God's plan,
arrived. In this theology, the "perfect" thing that arrived was the Scriptures. For many people in my denomination it is believed that with the
arrival of the Bible, there is no further need for certain spiritual gifts.

Yet, the apostle Paul made it very clear that apostles, prophets,
evangelists, and teachers are necessary for equipping the church, and
he told us these roles will be required for an extended, ongoing period
for the body of Christ on earth. Ephesians 4:11–13 does not give any
expiration date but rather indicates that these roles must continue so
the body of Christ is equipped and built up "until we all reach unity in
the faith and in the knowledge of the Son of God and become mature,
attaining to the whole measure of the fullness of Christ" (v. 13 NIV).

I don't believe the body of Christ has reached a level of unity, maturity, or fullness of Christ where we can say we don't need prophets and
apostles anymore or that certain gifts of the Spirit are not available
because they are not needed. For much of my life, I didn't really know
anything about the Holy Spirit other than the fact that I asked Jesus
into my heart and the Holy Spirit came in.

Then, as Rick and I began to become serious about moving into
full-time ministry, we started taking theology classes through our
Baptist church. One of the courses was called "Rightly Dividing" and
was based on the teachings of John Nelson Darby and C. I. Schofield,
pivotal figures in the development and popularization of dispensationalism.[1] I loved this course. It helped me to explain God because it

made everything tidy and less confusing. The operations of God were efficiently placed on a visual chart that was easily memorized. God was placed in boxes on the timeline chart; this is what he did and expected in each box of time. How wonderful it was to finally figure God out and have all the answers in hand! I could easily debate with my charismatic brethren because I was armed with theology that justified and explained why the supernatural gifts we saw in the New Testament had ceased.

My mother was even more of a hardliner than I was. Hundreds of volumes of theological books line the walls of her house. I know she's read them all because there is not a book that I have picked up that is not marked with her personal notes. She also has a lot of books on supernatural gifts, but I think the purpose was to fine-tune her arguments; the pages were lined with her contradictory objections backed by Scripture references.

I heard this preached from a pulpit of my former denominational church: "If your theology does not support your experience, then maybe you should rethink and change your theology." The comment was aimed at another denomination that believed in supernatural gifts, but looking back I see it was better fit with the doctrine of cessation that had blocked my own spiritual giftings for many years.

For every Scripture found to support the doctrine of cessation, there will be four other Scriptures that don't fit. And in order to make them work, we either change the definition of roles in the Bible, such as prophets and apostles, or change doctrines. The Bible never states that prophecy, healing, or tongues would cease after the apostles or New Testament era. In fact, Acts 2:17–18 suggests prophecy would continue: "In the last days, God says, I will pour out my Spirit on ALL people, your sons and daughters will prophesy, your young men will see visions, your old men will dream dreams." The apostle Paul told us to covet or earnestly desire to prophesy (1 Corinthians 14:1 NIV, emphasis mine).

In my childhood church, I was taught that prophecy is really just preaching, and although a preacher may have elements of prophecy and teaching in their message, Paul still differentiates it from teaching:

"And God has placed in the church first of all apostles, second prophets, third teachers, then miracles, then gifts of healing, of helping, of guidance, and of different kinds of tongues" (1 Corinthians 12:28 NIV).

Recently, my husband was at a conference focused around Christian business and listening to the Holy Spirit as an entrepreneur. The Holy Spirit pointed out a man in front of him and spoke to Rick, "I want you to tell that man that if he fixes the relationship with his wife, then I will bless his business." This would be a difficult message to deliver to a total stranger. Both Rick and I believe it's important to build relational equity before speaking something like this, but there are gentle ways we can do this if we choose respectful and kind words. Plus, Rick felt this was an immediate message from God.

Rick tapped the man on the shoulder and asked him if he was married with children. The man said, "No, I am divorced with children." This felt even more difficult for Rick, but now he knew he had heard the Holy Spirit correctly. If we are on the right track, we can trust the message will have its way. Rick gently continued, "I heard God say to me that your business took a toll on your marriage, but he is saying that if you will go and patch things up with your wife . . . whatever that means to you . . . God says he will bless your business." The man was stunned and couldn't respond.

The conference continued into the evening, and Rick didn't talk to the man again. The following day this same man came up to Rick with a smile on his face. "I came to this conference and didn't know why I came. I am Jewish, but today I received Jesus into my life." This is a good example of prophecy in action. Paul shows prophecy as revealing the secrets of someone's heart, leading them to fall down and worship God saying, "God is really among you!" (1 Corinthians 14: 24–25).

Having questions or uncertainty about Scripture results in debate. Debate turns into dogma, and dogma births doctrines, which form denomination structures. Denominations contain groups of "think-alikes." Staying within the confines of our denomination makes us feel safe and keeps us from challenging our belief system since everyone around us believes the same way. We become elite holders of the truth.

I get what denominational leaders are doing. They want to provide answers for their congregations to insulate them from questions that could become a slippery slope into apostasy. Questioning one's belief system can be tricky. Christians can feel a lot of guilt when they have questions, and leaders can contribute to that. What happens when our doctrinal belief system collides with life? It can lead to varied results: we create new theology or doctrinal beliefs, or we switch to different ones. Or we may start to question our entire belief system, which either causes us to develop deeper faith or walk away from Jesus. Sadly, too many former Christians have chosen this path, deconstructing their faith into nothingness. Just as I had hoped to hang a bag of packed red blood cells for my dying patient, God stands holding the bag of life, longing for each of us to engage in the healing waters of his river of life.

Rick and I began asking unwelcome questions at our little independent Baptist church. We noticed that the teaching was not lining up with the Bible. Even though this church taught us a lot about Scripture, the teaching on the gifts of the Holy Spirit, especially around prophecy, healing, and tongues, didn't seem consistent with the Bible. When our questions started, we were no longer welcome, and we started to experience abusive authoritative leadership. If we didn't adhere to the institutional rule books, we suffered shame, whether we inflicted it on ourselves out of guilt or felt it from the rest of the church. The atmosphere of the church became spiritually unhealthy to the point we had to accept the fact a new start was necessary.

We bought a home off the internet, sold most of our things, and loaded the rest of our stuff into a converted yellow school bus we had purchased to travel across the country to start over. The bus contained the last of our worldly goods, our five kids, and our dog. We looked like Jed Clampett and his crew from *The Beverly Hillbillies* driving down the road. Even the top of the bus was loaded with tons of stuff. Our children's friends from school wrote things all over the bus: peace symbols, autographs, and quotes. We were quite a sight as we roared out of town and sped down the highway to the other side of Canada, where Rick started university.

After years of cultish constraint, liberation should have been sweeter, but instead I teetered between the hysteric exhilaration of freedom and a fear of the unknown. While prohibited secular music blasted from the windows of the yellow bus and the past grew smaller in our rear-view mirror, the religious voices in my head were telling me I was on my way to hell. As we had expected, the church that had been a part of our lives for almost twenty years excommunicated us when we left, prohibiting any of their members to communicate with us. Our kids lost all their childhood friends.

If anyone is struggling to believe that the gifts of the Holy Spirit exist today, they may need to reevaluate the Scriptures and review their denominational teaching. Rick and I had to walk away from our theological roots and reevaluate the Scriptures for ourselves. This could not occur until we began to question what we had been taught. We pulled ourselves out of our religious denomination because of the questions we had around their doctrinal belief system, including their closed-door policy on the Holy Spirit.

I feel like the doctrine of cessation is a self-fulfilling prophecy. This doctrine creates a belief or expectation that influences the actual behavior of the entire congregation. In other words, by believing something will not happen, people unconsciously act in ways that bring about the predicted outcome. Even so, the Holy Spirit has a way of flowing through the most stubborn mindsets.

My father passed away a few years ago and my mother was struggling with loneliness and depression. This seemed to go on for several months, and I became deeply concerned about her health. It was during this time that I received a phone call from my sister. She seemed excited and cautious all at the same time. "Rhonda, something's happened to Mom. I think it's good, but she's not herself and I don't know what to think."

I couldn't contain my curiosity and called my mother. The person who answered the phone seemed unrecognizable to me. She excitedly began to tell me her story.

"When your father passed away, I struggled with loneliness. I just wanted my life to be over so that I could join him in heaven. Someone dropped off some DVDs from a church in the South hoping to encourage me. It was a Pentecostal church and as I watched I was struck by the joy they all seemed to have. I said to myself, 'I wonder if I'm missing something.' Two weeks later at two in the morning I woke up suddenly, sat bolt upright, and a heavenly language started coming out of my mouth. I couldn't stop it. When I did try to stop it, all I could say was, 'It's real! It's real! It's real!' and then it would start again. Rhonda, I am filled with so much joy. I wake up in the morning and the Holy Spirit speaks to me so clearly. I feel like I used to have access to God through 911 calls, but now I have a direct line."

As I listened to my mom, the staunch Baptist who would stand up in church and publicly oppose questionable doctrines associated with the charismatic movement, I began to laugh. The most hilarious part of this story is that the Holy Spirit chose to give my mother the gift of tongues that she had adamantly believed did not exist.

Our conversation ended with my mother now determined to publish abroad the deception of the "devilish" cessation doctrine that kept her from experiencing the fullness of the Holy Spirit.

Any denomination that does not teach the theology on the filling and fullness of the Holy Spirit can keep people in ignorance. New Christians or longtime Christians who have never been taught about the Holy Spirit or his gifts may not know they have this healing river that wants to flow out of them. They received Jesus as Savior and were born again. They feel his presence and know there has been a change inside but do not understand anything beyond this point. They may focus on spreading the gospel message, but the idea of a forceful flow of the Spirit through various gifts may seem frightening or foreign if this is not taught to them through a discipleship process. Theology can start or stop the River of Life.

CHAPTER 4
CONCEPT OF GOD

C hoosing to believe God still heals and that God is good was probably the most important foundation for my walk of faith. Is God good? We believed he was in the beginning when we turned to faith in him and asked him into our lives. But do we still believe he is good despite the sickness and suffering we encounter?

I saw this in myself—a form of sovereignty about God that morphed into fatalism. Do I believe that events such as sickness, suffering, famines, and wars are predetermined and inevitable? Or do I believe that God feels the same way we do about the pain and suffering in the world around us? Why did Jesus teach us to pray "Your will be done on earth as it is in heaven" (Matthew 6:10 NKJV) if the world's chaos is unavoidable or of no concern to God?

One of the greatest challenges to my concept of God occurred in 2010 while I was doing a community health internship in Haiti. There was a constant barrage of hungry people at my door asking for food or medical care. The local needs were so overwhelming and emotionally draining that we were advised to get away at least once a week.

On the weekends, many employees of foreign nonprofit or government organizations could be found at a hotel along the ocean near the city. It was an hour drive from our home, and we tried to go weekly to escape the misery around us. I had a love/hate relationship with this resort. Security guards and barriers surrounded the perimeter to keep out the locals. I hated the fact that I went there, but I longed for it as well. We paid our five dollars to use the facility for the beach and the restaurant. We could have a lovely meal and forget about suffering. Many guests at the hotel would numb their brain with excessive amounts of alcohol. It was a place of escape, a place where misery was not visible.

We arrived there one weekend with the same shameful, excited anticipation of a relaxing day at the beach. The sand was white, the sea sparkling blue. A gentle breeze caressed my body as I ran into a wave with a hop, a skip, and a jump. I floated on the ocean's surface, star-fished under the warmth of the sun. I whispered, "God, you are so good to me!"

I was not prepared for the question that answered my thankful burst of praise: "Rhonda, does that mean I am not good to the people on the other side of the fence?"

It was the closest experience I have had to hearing the audible voice of God. I choked and splashed my way to a standing position, the motion of the waves throwing me off balance. I had no answer for him. I could only stand there stunned by his blunt question. He was asking me what I believed about him, and he wanted an answer. I grappled with this question for more than a year.

In all honesty, I struggled to answer. Deep down in my soul I had unanswered questions about the traumatic experiences I had encountered in Haiti. I was miserable when we returned to Canada after the health internship. I was frustrated with the consumerism and materialism when so many other countries were struggling to meet physical needs. I became angry and argumentative with people who complained about government, healthcare, or basic first-world problems. They had no real needs and had no idea how good their lives were in Canada. I wanted to go back to Haiti; that was where I was needed. North America didn't need me.

I applied for several positions as a nurse practitioner in different organizations that would take me back into medical work in needy places, but God kept shutting doors. Opportunities opened in Canada, but I didn't want them. After several months of unemployment, I finally settled on a nurse practitioner job in Prince Edward Island (PEI), Canada. When I look back at this time in my life, I realize this job was exactly what I needed to heal from the trauma I had encountered during my time in Haiti.

The indigenous name for PEI is *Epekwitk*, which means "cradled in the waves." For me, PEI became a place of feeling cradled by God. This island cradled me and nurtured me back to life. More importantly, I was able to finally answer God's question, "Am I good to the people outside the fence?"—but it wasn't without gentle prodding.

I started to build a family practice in PEI and noticed a trend of mental health issues in my patient population. The beautiful, gentle island of *Anne of Green Gables* is not as idyllic as Lucy Maud Montgomery's dreamy descriptions. There was a sadness here for so many families struggling with unemployment. Often, one parent had to leave the family for employment thousands of miles away, enduring weeks if not months of separation in exchange for a steady paycheck. God began to speak to me about North America and foreign missionary work.

He highlighted the beautiful moments in Haiti. I reflected on the families who sat together outside at night without electricity, talking, laughing, playing games in the moonlight. God reminded me of the faith and love the Haitian people demonstrated, the way communities supported each other and sacrificed for each other in troubled times. Then God compared the strength of family, faith, and community in Haiti to the new patients I was encountering in my Canadian practice. He said gently, "Rhonda, in Haiti the people are rich in family, community, and faith, but they are poor in material goods and healthcare. Here in this place, people are rich in material goods and healthcare but have broken families, broken communities, and very little faith. You have been focusing on what you feel is more important, when the issues are just the opposite side of the same coin."

Finally, after almost a year waiting, God finally got his answer. Somehow, I had aligned the goodness of God with only one side of the coin. The side that included physical comforts, luxurious amenities, and easy solutions. I had come to the wrong conclusion about the needs of people. Once I saw the bigger picture of God's goodness, I knew. God is good to people on both sides. "Yes, God," I said. "You are entirely good."

Shortly after this revelation I became content and settled in my family practice in PEI. My frustration with consumerism and materialism was replaced with God's compassion toward broken people in broken communities with broken families. When the goodness of God is aligned with what we determine in our own thinking as good, we will invariably come to the wrong conclusions about the character of God.

What do we think about God? Has he told you about himself? I believe God longs to be understood. He longs for us to ask questions so that he can pull us deeper into seeing the world from his perspective.

First impressions can be difficult, and there have been times when I have formed opinions about an individual based on my first encounter. A bad first impression can be influenced by the opinions of others. I can push into the relationship for better understanding, or I can throw up suspicious boundaries while running the other way. Thankfully I am a listener and rarely form opinions about people unless I've spent the time necessary to hear their story.

Hearing someone's story is always a gamechanger for me. Reading or hearing secondhand information does not always give me a proper perspective of an individual. Understanding someone is found in intimacy, and intimacy between two people requires time, connection, and closeness. It often involves emotional, physical, and even spiritual bonding. Fostering intimacy requires trust, respect, communication, empathy, vulnerability, and even shared experiences.

I can read about my patient through previous medical records, opinions of specialists, and previous diagnoses, but I can come to conclusions that are not valid and miss the real reasons behind both physical and mental illness. It is the combination of information plus the physical encounter when I hear the patient's story from their own lips that helps me to know the individual in front of me.

I have a close friend whose husband is a judge. I deeply respect this man and have often said that if I ever had the misfortune of being dragged into court, I would want this man to be the judge. He is known as a man of integrity and honesty, and he works hard and serves his role with grace and incredible fairness.

I talked with my friend about her husband's role of judge and wondered how he dealt with this responsibility. She told me about one case that he needed to judge in the coming week. She described his desk loaded with files and papers regarding the individual who was being tried and told me that her husband asked for every piece of paperwork that could be found, from the early days in the foster system to every subsequent encounter with the law. He stayed in his office and studied this person's life so he could understand the challenges that were faced, the trauma the individual encountered, and any other social history that could shed light on the root causes that led to the crime. He felt that making a judgment balanced in justice and mercy could only be delivered through lengthy study and investigation of the life of the accused. Prior to the upcoming court case, he spent his weekend and days off poring over the life of one he would be required to pass judgment on in the following week.

One day I read a news article about my friend's husband. A complaint and accusation had made it into the local headlines about an unfair judgment in one of his cases. Despite a small public outcry, I knew this man's character was firm in fairness and integrity. His identity was based on delivering truth and justice in mercy. I never once questioned his actions, because I understood him at a different level than the public. Eventually truth prevailed and the accusations were silenced, but I am sure it must have been difficult for the judge to be maligned by the public for walking out his identity.

I see this as the same with God. He wants us to know who he is, and he longs to be understood. Many of us think God can handle it more than we can. Yes, he has broad shoulders to handle public opinion, but at the same time he longs for people to know him and understand him.

There have been so many times in my life when I have truly felt misunderstood and have tried to bring understanding to a situation to resolve a conflict or unfair judgment against me. I am not talking about when I am in the wrong and need to confess and apologize. I am talking about times when I have been judged by others for decisions I have made that were based on personal integrity and justice. It is so hurtful to be misunderstood by others and to hear secondhand gossip of what others are saying about you. I have found myself rambling on to another person, even oversharing information, so I can express my side of the story. The urgency within me that must explain itself is irresistible. *If only they knew me, they would understand my actions!* Being understood is a strong motivator for many of us. I think this is true because we are made in the image of God.

This longing to be heard, to be understood, to be known, comes from the heart of God. He speaks of this through the prophet Jeremiah:

> "Let the wise not boast of their wisdom or the strong boast of their strength or the rich boast of their riches, but let the one who boasts boast about this: that they have the understanding to know me, that I am the LORD, who exercises kindness, justice and righteousness on earth, for in these I delight," declares the LORD. (9:23–24 NIV)

I reflected on God's desire to be known while studying the story of Moses. The Bible says God "spoke to Moses face to face, as a man speaks with his friend" (Exodus 33:11 NKJV). While pondering this friendship with God, I heard God say to me, "Rhonda, I am tired of what people say about me. I would like people to understand me rather than just listen to secondhand information they hear from others." How much of our concept of God is based on a first impression or secondhand knowledge?

This friendship that Moses had with God was built on a desire to be known. Moses did a daring thing. He asked to see God. The conversation began with Moses saying things like "God, you're asking me to do things for you and you haven't even told me your name!" (see Exodus

33). Moses struggled with trust and self-confidence, and he began calling God out for asking him to do great things without having more information. Moses was going to step out and put himself on the line, but he needed more relational equity with God.

Have you ever been in a situation where you put your reputation on the line for someone or something that you weren't necessarily sure about? Moses needed proof, and God's answers were not enough for him. Moses basically said, "I'm done with talking! I need to see proof. Now show me your glory" (see Exodus 33:18). This was a big ask. No one could see the face of God and live, but God put proper safety measures in place, and as he passed by Moses, he shouted out a proclamation about himself that he wanted Moses to understand. God speaks his identity statement: "The LORD, the LORD God, merciful and gracious, longsuffering and abounding in goodness and truth, keeping mercy for thousands, forgiving iniquity and transgression and sin, by no means clearing the guilty, visiting the iniquity of the fathers upon children's children to the third and the fourth generation" (Exodus 34:6–7 NKJV). There are so many characteristics that God shouts out in his expression of himself, but its entirety can be summarized in the following three statements:

1. I am good.
2. I am merciful.
3. I will judge bad things that people do.

The basis to intimacy with another individual is understanding who they are. Moses asked to see God's glory. Glory is often described as a radiant manifestation of God's physical presence, but when he showed his glory to Moses it was more than this; it was his physical presence combined with his identity statement.

Failing to understand his identity will lead to improper conclusions about who God is and why he does or does not do something we think he should. Many people refuse to come to God, or they walk away from God, because they sit in judgment of his character. Ultimate intimacy is found in trusting that he is good when we think he isn't, that he is merciful when we think he shouldn't be, and that he has or will bring judgment eventually when we think he should step in right now.

My struggle with God's identity statement occurred when I was faced with extreme poverty in a developing nation. The test of faith occurs in the dirty ditches of life. You encounter the *real* in the dirty ditches. Real smells, real sounds, real emotional agony, real helplessness, real dialogue. All this *real* brings forth questions for God. The dirty ditches of life are where the hard questions are asked and conclusions about the character of God are made.

Choosing to believe God is good, merciful, and just amid the constant irritating hurtful jabs from our experiences in life is hard work. This is why we're told to labor to enter into rest (Hebrews 4:11). Faith is hard work. Faith is laborious. It is much easier to be faithless.

I work in a faith-based nonprofit healthcare clinic. Broken and struggling people back up their dump trucks to my exam rooms, and I hear the warning sounds of the backup beepers. They wait with bated breath, hand on the dump lever for the moment they can alleviate their burden by dumping their pain onto me, the ready listener. Some of these patients are brilliant, well-educated leaders within their professional fields, but their inner emotional pain has borne the fruit of disease. When I try to assess their spirituality and ask leading questions like "Do you believe in prayer?", I can see immediate irritation on their faces and receive logical explanations as to why they do not believe in a god. On occasion I empathize with their struggles to believe in a good God, nod my head in agreement, and say, "Yes, I know. It's not easy to believe. Having faith is hard work. It's easier to not believe when we see a world that is crumbling all around us." This usually stumps these elite, successful, high-achievers who were good at everything in life. The idea of getting a D in faith confuses them.

When the disciples came to Jesus to ask him the specifics of their job description, they asked, "What must we do, to be doing the works God requires?" Jesus answered, "This is the work of God, that you believe in the one he has sent" (John 6:28–29). For those outside of a life of faith, Christianity can appear weak and brainless, but the Christian walk of faith means choosing to believe despite all odds and walking forward in hope. This means I continue to pray for the impossible and not just for the possible.

There was a time when I didn't know how to pray for the impossible. That was before I learned how much God longs for people to know him and understand him. Before I realized the Holy Spirit is the river of healing. Before I met others who were already experiencing the flow.

LEARNING FROM OTHERS

I have been a nurse since 1986 and became a nurse practitioner in 2010. I still go home after a long shift wondering if I did the right thing. Did I get the right diagnosis? Did I prescribe the right medicine? The biggest lesson I have learned in my profession as a nurse practitioner is that I will always be a lifelong learner who will never know it all.

My first mentor in healthcare was a family physician in Prince Edward Island, Canada. His name was Dr. Meek—and he was so true to his name. He was renowned in his community for being the "best doctor ever!" and had a national award to prove it. When I started my first family practice, he said these words and I have not forgotten them: "Rhonda, the first forty years are the hardest." We practice medicine based on rigorous scientific research and evidence, but we still practice. We try medical treatments in faith that those who tried them before us had good results.

A spiritual practice is no different. By faith we take the truth of the Scriptures and practice them. Whether it's walking out my medical or spiritual authority, I walk forward humbly by faith on the shoulders of giants. I am so thankful for my Baptist heritage and the people who built a strong foundation in the Scriptures. I am also grateful for the spiritual mentors I encountered in the Baptist church in Edmonton, Alberta, who mentored us in a safe place where we could stir up our spiritual gifts that were not yet realized or practiced (the same ones who prayed for the young pastor who was healed from hepatic cancer).

Our initial introduction to this group occurred in 2015. We had just moved to Alberta from Prince Edward Island and began attending Central Baptist Church in Edmonton. It was difficult to get to know people, so we joined a weekend course in hopes of growing closer to this church community. During that weekend, a group of men prayed over my husband. A man named Greg laid his hands on him and described a picture he was seeing that only God could have known. Later, I asked Rick to point Greg out to me. I wanted to know more.

Was this the gift of prophecy? Was he a prophet? The very word was confusing, and my theology barred me from challenging my Baptist heritage. I walked closely with God. I heard Him—His kind voice spoke in my spirit through the Scriptures—but pictures? Absolutely not. This was totally off limits, opening us to all kinds of demonic influence. Or so I thought.

I stood there looking at Greg. The echo of his words to Rick were hammering through a walled-off area in my spirit and now there was a breach. Light began pouring onto a gift that lay dormant.

Rick introduced me to Greg, and I learned he wasn't the only one. He represented a small underground group in this Baptist church that had been honing their prophetic giftings for over seventeen years. They met weekly and prayed for people by appointment only. This was a protected membership, a closed group by special invitation only. Now I was intrigued.

I understood why it was this way. There had been hurt in the past. Word got out in this church about the mysterious activities within this small group, and some of their members were pulled before the elders of the church for questioning and a "trying of the spirits." Honestly, I got where those elders were coming from, because I was cut from the same theological cloth. I had spent a great deal of time poring over the Scriptures to fine-tune my doctrinal arguments.

I learned that the Holy Spirit always comes bearing gifts. These gifts are upgrades that we are given to bless his church and build the kingdom of God. Some of these gifts are listed in various portions of the Scriptures, such as 1 Corinthians 12, Romans 12, and Ephesians 4. Some of us don't know we have gifts from the Holy Spirit, some of us have been taught to hide them, some of us don't know how to use them, and some of us deny these gifts even exist. This last one is where I used to firmly park my beliefs.

But there was something about the prophetic prayer Rick had experienced, and I wanted to be a part of whatever this was. How could I get in? How could I learn more?

I discovered I could schedule a session for personal prayer, so I immediately booked an appointment for both of us. That prayer time jackhammered away any remaining resistance and pulled Rick and me into the light of prophecy. We came away from that evening like we had just emerged from a tight cocoon; we were shaking out our wings and about to fly. Even better still, by unanimous decision, we received an invitation to join the group. We were crossing the theological line of our denominational roots and running after forbidden fruit. Our lives were about to change.

We moved from Canada to Hawaii the next year. Rick and I had already been in missions for several years when we felt a call to join YWAM, which was based in Kailua Kona, Hawaii. We began Discipleship Training School in 2016 at the advice of the pastor of our church in Canada, who was a former YWAM leader from Scotland and well acquainted with the organization.

During my second week of Discipleship Training School, I was literally hit with the love of God. The common corporate area for gathering of staff and students is called the Ohana Court. The place was packed with over six hundred people listening attentively to an honest and challenging message echoing across this space from a woman speaking on God's love.

She began to shout out that God's love is not biased. If he loves everyone, then this is the type of love we should have as well. The challenge in my heart came when she started to drop names of Christian leaders I personally disliked. She went on to say that she loved well-known Christian leaders who were theologically opposed to one another. "I love them all!" she proclaimed.

I sat in my seat and mumbled to myself, "I don't love those guys." The comment in my mind came from denominational prejudice. And that is when it happened. A wave of overwhelming energy came across the Ohana Court and hit me in my chest. The only example I can compare it to is the time I had to go to the emergency room and was given a shot of epinephrine because of an anaphylactic reaction to a medication.

Adrenaline is not pleasant; in fact, it can be quite frightening. Your heart feels like it's about to explode in your chest; your eyesight is so keen and rapid that it is difficult to see, especially with bright fluorescent lights in the ER; your hearing is superpowered; and your body feels like a jet engine and the pilot has just pulled the thruster for takeoff.

While everyone else was listening to the message, I was completely weighed down in my chair, immoveable, trying to open my eyes but the light was blinding. My voice could only quietly call out helplessly to Rick who stood beside me, "God marked me with his love, Rick. . . . He marked me. . . . I can't move. I can't see!" I felt the presence of God in an intensely powerful, personal way. I had never in my life felt the heaviness or fire of the Holy Spirit like this. It felt strange, even slightly scary, but at the same time I sensed an overwhelming sensation of love and comfort. I felt completely safe in his presence.

I don't know any other way to describe this. I had never experienced anything like this in my life like this up to that point. I think I had felt the heaviness in prayer and even felt anguish of intercession, but never the fire of the Spirit, which is really the love of God. I walked around with a weighted blanket of peace for three days.

The supportive community of experienced prophets in Alberta who met on Mondays had facilitated a safe, comfortable prophetic mentorship for Rick and me. They had built a prophetic team that quietly and humbly utilized their gifts as a working group that covertly edified the local church. It was in Canada that Rick and I stirred up our gift of prophecy in a safe, healthy training environment. Success was celebrated and missteps were coached. There were no prophetic clones here, and I believe the strength of this group was found in the individuality of each member and the unique way prophecy was demonstrated. This safe space allowed the Holy Spirit to teach individuals to see, hear, demonstrate, and live out their prophetic gift in authentic uniqueness in a close-knit community of prophets.

Then God led us to Kona where he immersed me in his love, deepening my understanding of his ways and opening me to further healing. My experience with the intense love of God led to uncovering the guilty root of brokenness in my life that had been caused by my brother's accident.

As more and more children of God are birthed into the kingdom, the body of Christ should be welcoming these new novices just like the fictional character Professor Xavier from the movie *X-Men*. This professor recognizes the supernatural gifts of individuals who are called "mutants" by society. These gifted individuals are often broken and hurt. They live isolated lives and are misunderstood, even ostracized or imprisoned by the forces in the world wanting to maintain control or dominion. Professor Xavier recognizes that these gifted individuals need a place to be accepted and affirmed. They often need family and a sense of belonging, so he builds the School for Gifted Youngsters.

Likewise, churches should serve as havens and training grounds for the children of God in ways of the Holy Spirit, offering education and support so we can all edify the church and learn how to utilize our special gifts. In this setting, the River of Life is free to flow.

CHAPTER 5
GOING WITH THE FLOW

Denial ain't just a river in Egypt.
MARK TWAIN

I am a gamer. A video gamer. I picked up gaming during COVID at the age of sixty. I reached for my husband's Xbox controller as a desperate measure to escape boredom during quarantine. My husband couldn't watch me play; my erratic use of the controller made him dizzy and nauseous. With time, I mastered an older role-playing game and eventually one of the most difficult video games of 2023. After hours of play I reached high levels in this game that even impressed my son who is a seasoned gamer.

Not long ago I found a game that I can play online with my children. After a busy day of seeing clients, I unwind by gaming. It's fun, it's good for my brain, and it gives me time with my kids. It is a player-versus-player game that requires a lot of quick thinking, moving, and utilization of weapons. Every few months the map changes and new weapons are added. Recently a water-bending weapon was added, which has become my all-time favorite. A circle of water surrounds my character's waistline and shoots from the belly with precision and accuracy.

I'll be honest, there have been days when I have spent so much time gaming that when I leave the house and see something in the real world that reminds me of the game, my mind thinks it's still gaming. These reactions in the real world remind me that I have spent far too much time gaming that day.

A truth can be pulled from this vulnerable, self-revealing illustration. Gaming in an imaginary virtual world links me to a physical action on a controller. Can we spend so much time with Jesus that it spills over into our physical world? I have been spending more and more time with Jesus lately, and I will be the first to tell you: Yes. The more time we spend with Jesus, the more he becomes a part of our daily life.

TEA TIMES WITH JESUS

There are certain words that can cause discomfort for Christians. We approve of the word *meditation* because it's in the Bible. Plus, David meditated, so it must be okay. But the word *imagination* is often associated with being evil, and there is cautionary biblical teaching associated with its use.

As a child I sang about the river of life, yet I couldn't grasp its reality. Several rivers are mentioned in the Bible, and often they were associated with life, blessing, judgment, or geographical landmarks. In Genesis 2 we read about the rivers Pishon, Gihon, Tigris, and Euphrates that flowed out of the garden of Eden. The Nile River plays a significant role in the life of Moses, including being turned to blood during the plagues (Exodus 7:20).

One of the most prominent rivers is the Jordan River, which served as a boundary to the Promised Land (Joshua 3:14–17). Elijah and Elisha crossed it just before Elisha was taken up to heaven in a chariot of fire (2 Kings 2:8–14). The Jordan is also significant because it is the river where John the Baptist baptized Jesus. There is a river called the River of Life located in heaven. It flows from the throne of God and symbolizes a flow of water that brings healing to the nations (Revelation 22:1–2).

Rivers carry deep theological, historical, and spiritual significance throughout the Bible. Some of these rivers have a sort of mystical power that we long for. We are like Indie in *Indiana Jones and the Kingdom of the Crystal Skull*. We believe this river of life can only be found through dangerous, death-defying jungle adventures and years of archaeological expertise. We know it's there. We see evidence of its power, but access to this life-giving drink seems impossible, unbelievable, or even a superstitious myth. Our belief system simply won't allow us to go with the flow. At least mine didn't.

My theology gave imagination a bad rap. It focused on Scriptures that called the imagination evil (Genesis 6:5) and said that every imagination of man's heart is evil (Genesis 8:21). Jeremiah 7:24 ties an imagination of their evil heart to rebellion. I was taught that I was supposed to "cast down" my imagination like it says in 2 Corinthians 10:5. I spent a lot of time erecting fences within my mind. I cast down all imagination and would not allow myself to even imagine Jesus, because that would mean I was creating my own image of God.

However, when King David said, "I have set the LORD always before me; because he is at my right hand, I will not be shaken" (Psalm 16:8), how did David set the Lord before him and see him at his right hand? This required imagination, right? And if so, does that make it real?

There are several places in the Bible where Jesus repeatedly employed metaphors, a communication skill he used often while he lived on earth. He called his body bread (John 6:35), he called himself the Good Shepherd (John 10:11), and he compared himself to a vine (John 15:5) and a gate (John 10:8). Metaphors are essential for our imagination. They take complex ideas and connect them with things we can see, hear, feel, or experience in the real world. Jesus wants to utilize our imagination so we can see in our minds the spiritual truths he is trying to convey. Imagination is the movie screen in our life where we can see and hear from God in the realm of the kingdom. It is where our faith seems to begin. It is the place where we can see and hear the reruns of old episodes from the past so that our faith does not waver in the present.

I am not sure if everyone's process is the same as mine, but when I read the Bible I see the words in my imagination. If there are metaphors, I immediately see the comparison of what is conveyed. When I read about Jesus calling himself the living water, I imagine him with outstretched hands holding water, and I can see myself drinking out of his hands.

The movie screen captures audio as well, and this is where I hear God's voice. Imagination is not faith, but it is a place where faith can ignite, a place that needs to be activated, fostered, controlled, and renewed so that faith can rise and act.

I sometimes have difficulty understanding or comprehending God the Father, God the Son, and God the Holy Spirit, but when I think about God's ingenuity and wisdom in coming back to earth in a holy spiritual form, I get *wow* moments that leave me reeling with wonder.

One of these *wow* moments occurs when I think about Jesus telling his disciples that he had to leave. He basically says, "Guys, if I don't leave you and go up to be with my Father, then I won't be able to return to all of you in the form of the Holy Spirit." Jesus was limited in his physical form on earth. He was only able to minister to a select group of people in a select geographical location at one time, but the Holy Spirit, who is God in Spirit form, can minister to whoever, wherever, whenever, 24/7.

When we invite him into our lives, he brings life with him, and we are reborn spiritually within our physical bodies. From this point forward, the beautiful Holy Spirit becomes our guide, our comforter, our lover, and our friend, and he partners with us and flows out of our lives to those around us. The flow is his power, not ours.

I experience many close times with Jesus in what I refer to as "tea times." These are special times I set aside for encounters with the Holy Spirit. As I quiet myself in prayer and let my mind open to hear and see Jesus, in my imagination I usually find him in some special place where he has prepared tea and a treat. Of course I can't physically drink the tea or eat the snacks, but the setting invites me in for intimate conversation with Jesus. We discuss life, and our time together is always vivid and memorable. And good.

In the Old Testament, the prophet Asaph speaks the word of the Lord in Psalm 81:10: "I am the LORD thy God which brought thee up out of the land of Egypt: open thy mouth wide, and I will fill it" (KJV). David writes, "Oh taste and see that the LORD is good" (Psalm 34:8). Jesus says, "I am the bread of life; whoever comes to me shall not hunger, and whoever believes in me shall never thirst" (John 6:35). These verses leave us with a picture of consuming bread and water. John 6:63 explains that it is Jesus's words that are to be consumed because they are spirit and they are life: "It is the Spirit who gives life; the flesh profits nothing. The words that I speak to you are spirit, and they are life" (NKJV).

I am notorious for forgetting to eat food throughout the day. Sometimes I make myself pause, sit, and eat because otherwise I start feeling faint. This also occurs for us spiritually. We may not get the same physical symptoms of becoming physically tired and weak, but the symptoms of spiritual depletion are there. Faith, like physical energy, becomes faint, and we can even lose our thirst and desire for spiritual things. When we take the time to pause and eat and drink, the energy of faith keeps us running the race that is set in front of each one of us.

Pausing and listening for Jesus to speak is like waiting for a big dripping spoonful of honey. The prophets Ezekiel and John described visions of eating a scroll of God's Word and tell us it tasted like honey (Ezekiel 2:8–3:3; Revelation 10:9–11). The prophet David also gives us the same mouthwatering imagery when he tells us that God's words are sweeter than honey and the drippings of the honeycomb (Psalm 19:10). Jesus uses various means to speak to me, but I must admit that I prefer his voice.

His words feed my spirit. His words are the vital force that sustains me and flows from me. The flow of the Holy Spirit can be like the flow of water: it comes from high places where there is higher pressure to lower places in the earth.

The following vision is a revelatory account of a moment I had with Jesus during one of our tea times. The encounter left its mark on me, affirmed me as a medical professional, and called me higher to take authority over my profession.

THE VISION

I hadn't been to this place before. There was nothing but sand dunes and a dried-up riverbed that ran through the low crevices on a curvy horizon. I was surprised by my clothing. It was so simplistic: a breezy one-piece linen robe pulled over my head and hanging loosely just above my ankles. There was a belt around my waist with a small leather pouch that hung on my left side. *So medieval*, I mused. Only a slight, occasional breeze swept across the hot landscape, picking up some dust and swirling it across my face.

Water had flowed here once before. The trail of rocks and gravel, covered with layers of dry sand, wound through the low valleys between the sand dunes. I could trace its winding pathway through this desert place into the distance. To my right was an old, weathered rowboat that had obviously been abandoned and had seen better days. It seemed sound enough sitting half in the riverbed and half lodged into the sandy bank.

What is this place? I didn't usually meet Jesus for our tea times in places like this. Sometimes it was under the same pear tree back on The Hill where I would sit with my grandfather for lunch. Other times our setting was in a rose garden or on a dock by a lake. I can usually spot Jesus or at least find a path that is highlighted so that I can find my way to him, but not here. This was unlike any other meeting place, so I stood there waiting. I called his name but was only answered by the sound of wind stirring up the sand in front of my feet.

And then I heard it. Just a gurgle at first, seeming to come from a group of stones amid the riverbed about twenty feet to my right. And then I saw it. Small bubbles of water mixed with dusty dirt emerged from the stones. Suddenly, the timid, joyful, bubbling spring began to cough and hack forceful bursts of water into the dry, thirsty riverbed floor. I looked at the derelict boat and felt the cool water pool around my ankles and wet the hem of my robe. I instinctively climbed into the boat. I thought I would need to do some real tugging to dislodge it from the sand, but the water was coming incredibly fast, so I let buoyancy do the work.

The dried riverbed and the sudden coughing cacophony of bubbling, gurgling water filled me with questions. What was the dry riverbed? I could trace its impression through the dunes by its subtle winding path of soft mounds hiding jagged rocks and debris beneath layers of sand. I couldn't help but wonder, *Why did the flow of water stop in the first place and why did it suddenly emerge from the ground beside me?* In the past, the derelict wooden rowboat had obviously floated on the water's surface. I had a lot of questions for Jesus, but there were certain aspects of the vision that were clear to me. Once upon a time there was a river. It had dried up. It was flowing again and was carrying me to Jesus.

It didn't take long. The dry riverbed transformed itself into a powerful river, and I was picked up and carried along like a leaf. The river knew where to go. This was familiar territory to the flow of water, and as the mounting sound of rushing water moved across the desert, it was followed by the grateful sigh of a satisfied parched and thirsty riverbed.

I could see something in the distance—a large, white building to the east beyond the sand dunes, with mountains rising behind. I could tell the river was naturally winding toward this place. Maybe this was where I would meet him? I relaxed my back against the side of the rowboat. It was taking me to where he would be.

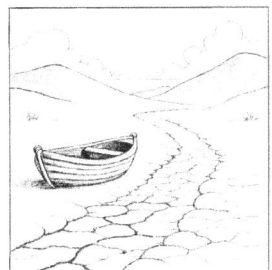 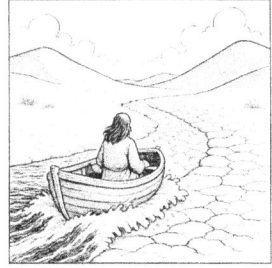 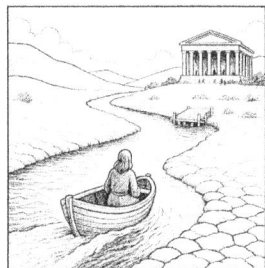

I should have known. It was always this way. Sometimes I could find him quickly, other times I would need to search or wait for some sort of clue, but he never failed to meet with me. Today I was letting the river do the work. It would lead me to him.

I was moving quickly now, and the building in the distance was coming closer. I could see an old wooden dock jutting up from the sand. The river would soon rush by, and I knew I would have to try to grab onto the dock before the force of the river pulled me past. I was supposed to go into that building. That was where he would be.

The current of the river was so powerful now that I felt like I was riding a wave with my derelict boat. The river turned to the left, flinging my boat to the right. I watched as the river's tidal wave slammed into the dock's weathered pylons about a hundred yards in front of me. This was going to be tricky. I prepared to grab the edge of the dock, and as my little boat veered toward the wooden edge, I managed to grab a post and hold firm until I clumsily rolled myself onto the dock. Once my weight left the boat, the small vessel veered forward, was tossed into the foamy swirling current, and rounded the bend out of sight.

I sat for a moment and examined my surroundings. The sound of rushing water had subsided, the river now deep and peaceful. The white building reminded me of a Greek Parthenon, its once-white stone exterior covered with dusty grime, but I could tell it had once been a grandiose and stately structure.

Six or seven priestlike individuals, all dressed like me, were working in the sparse dry fields outside the building. They were feverishly hoeing their small garden plots in poor, stony soil that appeared to yield very little greenery. It seemed an incredible amount of work for such little return. Each one worked in isolation and seemed unaware of each other's struggle to bring forth fruit from the dry, rocky earth. As I walked past them, they didn't acknowledge me. I knew where I needed to go, and I instinctively moved toward the Greek-looking building.

Huge pillars on the porch loomed upward, and as I walked up the stairs I could feel a cool breeze flowing from the darkened entrance. I was in awe. This place was huge and majestic, and I felt small as I walked quietly into the vast space. The cool floor shone glossy like a mirror. I thought it might be marble, but it was gray and solid like granite. Tall walls were lined with beautifully carved wooden bookshelves that rose to the ceiling roughly fifty feet high. Books, parchments, scrolls, and almost every type of written material filled the shelves. There was not a space on any wall that did not contain some written information, but the majority were books—old books, beautifully covered books, leather books, tattered books, thick books, and thin books. It was beautiful and overwhelming all at the same time.

Somehow, deep within my spirit I knew this place contained the world's collection of medical knowledge. This place stored every piece of medical research, as well as medical case studies, experiments, trials, statistics, medicinal compounds, and herbal recipes. I felt incredibly humbled and small in this place.

My gaze fell to the middle of the building. I could see Jesus in the distance sitting in a straight-backed, throne-like chair. I knew he would be here. I didn't run to him like I usually do. This moment seemed too serious. I felt like I was standing in a thick cloud of heaviness, the weightiness of what I sensed as a physical manifestation of wisdom and knowledge that permeated this place. Despite the weightiness of my surroundings, I walked forward to the One in the center of the room. He didn't speak but I could hear his voice in my spirit.

"Rhonda, everything in this place is good. It is wisdom from above, but remember to keep me at the center."

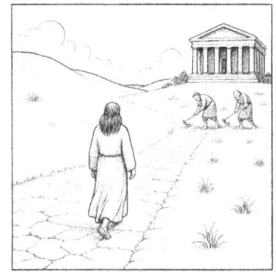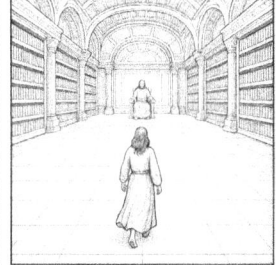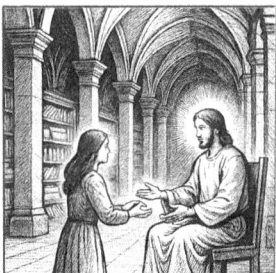

I looked down again at my priestlike robe that matched those worn by the people working outside in the dry, barren soil. Was I one of those poor individuals, dressed in priestly robes, gardening their small dry patches of vegetables, bringing forth very little fruit? How many of us in healthcare find ourselves here? We do the best we can with what we have. We apply our training and utilize our resources, but in the meantime there is a river of healing that God wants to release through us. And in that moment I understood. I was given a priestly role as a healthcare professional.

I was part of a medical priesthood. I was a priest on this earth, holding education and knowledge in one hand and the divine in the other. I was meant to open a gate so a powerful river of life could flow once again. I also realized this vision was not meant only for me. It is for anyone called into the profession of healthcare—even those priests outside working their dry, fruitless garden patches.

Trembling before Jesus, I walked forward and said, "I cannot do this without you. I need you to touch my hands so that I can release healing to the world around me." It was there in that magnificent place that I found my identity. I was called to repair a breach that had occurred between medicine and the supernatural. I reached out my hands and he knowingly smiled and complied. I think he did this just to reassure me. We both knew I already had this spiritual gift. It was just ragged and hidden beneath years of painful discouragement, skepticism, and hopelessness. It was time for the river to flow again. It was time to stir up my God-given gifts.

Standing before Jesus in the medical hall of fame surrounded by a library of the worlds' collection of research and wisdom affirmed me of a few things: he was pleased with me as a nurse practitioner, and medical science and wisdom are good, but Jesus is at the center of it all.

I reflected on that vision for months, encouraged. I realized that everything I had worked for—years of education and clinical experience, hundreds of hours of researching evidence and the study of current treatments—was *good*. I had followed him when he called me into nursing and then back to graduate school to become a family nurse practitioner. It all provided a strong foundation for the Holy Spirit to flow through me to bring hope and healing to others.

When we invite Jesus into our life, he delightfully accepts the invite and the Holy Spirit—who is Jesus himself—runs enthusiastically into our body with incredible joy. He lives within us and does not use us like a robot or like someone possessed by an alien force. He partners with us, providing us with the life-giving force of his Spirit so that we can live as champions within a world of chaos and sickness. The Holy Spirit lives in us, and his power flows outward from the center of who we are to advance God's kingdom.

I know now why the belly water-bender is my favorite weapon in my newest video game. It represents the powerful flow of the Holy Spirit that Jesus foretold, the living water that flows forth "out of his belly" in healing. When I find myself praying for a medical situation, imagining the river flowing from my belly helps me to see it in my mind.

The trustworthy authority of John 7:37 and the visual picture of the metaphor leads to increased faith. Faith then leads to physical action and partnership with the Holy Spirit, which enables the flow of power through me and the unique gifts that have been given to me. The outflow of the Holy Spirit is unique to each one of us and may occur through a gift of wisdom, prophecy, healing, or miracles.

Can you pause here for a moment and imagine a forceful river flowing from your belly? There is so much power in pausing and partnering with the Holy Spirit. We can imagine a forceful river of life bursting from our belly and sending life-giving power to whoever and whatever is situated within our radius of influence. And it all flows from the center—from Jesus. As is said of Jesus, "Out of his belly shall flow rivers of living water" (John 7:37 KJV), so it is for us.

Living, healing waters. Flowing. Through the Holy Spirit and through us.

CHAPTER 6
EDUCATION IS GOOD

The whole purpose of education is to turn mirrors into windows.
SIDNEY J. HARRIS

I graduated in 1986 with a two- to three-year college-level diploma, the requirement for entry to practice as a registered nurse at the time. It wasn't until the 1990s that nursing moved toward an undergraduate degree. Eventually, entry to practice required a university-level nursing education—while grandfathering older existing diploma nurses into nursing practice.

What followed should have been expected: healthcare facilities became battlefields between the old and the new. The old felt the threat of the new. The old criticized the new for their lack of practical training. The new questioned the old. Hunched-over bed makers jostling urinals and bedpans were puzzled and frustrated at these young, confident newbies with excellent posture. New theories and talk of evidence-based practice spread like irritation in hospital hallways. I watched this conflict with interest.

I didn't join the group of mumbling patriots complaining about their low back pain. I appreciated the fresh wave of knowledge and confidence that came onto the floor with these young nurses. They were changing old practices that needed necessary upgrades and revising outdated guidelines that proved worthless and sometimes even harmful to patients.

Around this time I went to an educational session at my workplace and watched a short video titled *Who Moved My Cheese?*, based on a book of the same name by Dr. Spencer Johnson.[1] The book is a brief tale of two mice and two humans who live in a maze. Every day they go to the same place in the maze for their cheese, until one day they are faced with change. Their cheese has been moved. The book tells us that change is inevitable and encourages us to anticipate, adapt, monitor, and enjoy change because it will happen again.

This was the final straw for me. I applied for the post-RN Bachelor of Nursing program and joined this new stream of nurses. I became a traitor to the old. One of my colleagues accused me of being selfish. During a tiresome nightshift she snarled at me, "You should be saving your money for your children's education!" I ignored her. My cheese had already been moved. It was the year 2000 and I was working part-time at a local hospital, my children were in elementary school, and Rick and I were in the middle of a renovation project. Despite what seemed like poor timing, I applied for the Bachelor of Nursing program and began the journey toward a degree in nursing.

One of the first courses in the program was Nursing 311, taught by an older, well-spoken nursing educator. Based on critical thinking, the course altered my personal biases and released me into the academic world. The instructor basically described it like this: "The definition of critical thinking is thinking about your thinking so that you can think better." Even though I was college educated and had graduated as a registered nurse a few years earlier, I did not necessarily understand the concept of critical thinking.

At the time, we were attending the small independent Baptist church we eventually had to leave. Unlike the other wives in this church, I worked outside the home. Nursing was one profession that seemed to be acceptable for a woman. There was a strong emphasis on homeschooling, home births, avoiding birth control, and natural foods. I became a huge granola mom. I sincerely wanted the best for my family, and my circle of influence was other granola moms in our church who were hyper-fixated on warding off the world's evils found in food, medicine, education, and philosophy. It requires a great deal of energy to live with a perspective of impending doom.

Nursing 311 opened a new lens and changed my outlook of the future. I went from a defensive doom-and-gloom backyard bunker thinker to a seeker of spiritual offense that would create scoring opportunities for Team Kingdom. Being able to think critically launches you from the grip of religious tradition, rigid self-imposed rules, group conformity, the fear of man, and impending doom. God is a big thinker, and his ways are high above ours.

There was another significant course that stared me down on the path to my Bachelor of Nursing degree. In this course I was introduced to the dragon I would need to slay. His name was Statistics. If you couldn't defeat this monster, you were doomed to failure. The statistics monster became the talk of legends. I left this course for the very last. But critical thinking and statistics are foundational to science, and if we are real seekers of truth who want to make the world a better place, then we should be good scientists—even if that includes statistics. So I faced the monster and made it to the other side. I proudly graduated with a Bachelor of Nursing degree.

Higher education is exactly that—it is higher, and it requires mental aerobics and training to reach it. At the same time, we can receive wisdom and guidance through Bible knowledge and spiritual insight from the Holy Spirit. Solomon wrote about wisdom crying in the streets, "Hey! Are there any takers? I have valuable knowledge, guidance readily available!" We need both. But that's a more difficult collaboration than trying to get old nurses and young nurses to agree on how to use bedpans.

The scientific academic world has a difficult relationship with the church. This is not new. History reminds us of early thinkers like Galileo, who is called the father of modern science.[2] He proposed that the sun, not the earth, was the center of the universe. In 1633 he was placed on trial by the Catholic Church as a heretic, forced to recant, and sentenced to house arrest for the remainder of his life. All of his works were banned. Giordano Bruno expanded on the same teaching and suffered the same fate.[3] He was arrested, spent seven years in prison, and was burned at the stake in Rome for heresy. Copernicus was able to avoid persecution because he released his work on his deathbed.[4]

Medicine is a science that pushes boundaries and can seem like an egotistical know-it-all in the room. Medicine can be healing, it can be comforting, it can be intimidating, it can be proud and elite, it can puff us up, it can humble us, it can be corrupt, and it can be miraculous. These contradictory conclusions have a profound effect on our opinions about pursuing higher education, about research and what we believe about the science of medicine. When I become skeptical, suspicious, proud, and elite and think I have a medical answer to a spiritual problem, I remember my vision with Jesus when he said, "All of this is good, but keep me at the center."

Several Christians throughout history have made significant contributions to science, such as Gregor Mendel, an Augustinian friar who is often called the "father of modern genetics," and Antoine van Leeuwenhoek, a devout Dutch Christian often referred to as the "father of microbiology." But something has happened in the church, especially in our Western world. The academic scientific world is viewed with suspicion and contempt, and there is a general pervading view that higher education is a slippery slope into apostasy. This Christian mindset constructs a false barrier to higher education and can lead to dangerous consequences.

I was speaking with a leader of a Christian missionary organization who felt that as an organization, we were sending ill-equipped missionaries. "We are sending illiterate people without skills as missionaries to the nations," he said. Christian clichés like "God doesn't call the qualified, he qualifies the called" can be misconstrued and place an unbalanced emphasis on spiritual development associated with ministry within the church. God needs his people to discover their identity, their gifts, and their calling, and then he needs us to develop our knowledge and skills to enter every sphere of society and build the kingdom of God. Jesus asks us to go into the world and make disciples. This word *disciples* is often associated with spiritual development, but I believe it also applies to professional and vocational training.

Every year I mentor nurse practitioner students and play a part in launching them into the healthcare industry. It is my hope that I am not just transmitting knowledge, but also cultivating values and behaviors that will influence healthcare. Effective discipleship requires two things: a mentor and a learner. The mentor has something valuable sought after by the learner, and this leads to a place of training and influence. Jesus calls us to make disciples; how can we do this if we have not prepared ourselves so that we have something to offer?

My husband and I have served in several different Christian organizations. Our most recent volunteer journey was in 2018 with YWAM, aboard a medical ship that delivered healthcare to isolated areas in the world. I served as a nurse practitioner in Papua, New Guinea, for nine months. It was incredibly challenging and physically demanding to deliver aid in extremely difficult circumstances to some of the most isolated places on earth.

When our ship anchored in a community located in West New Britain, we were met with tribal regalia and celebration. Not only did our ship carry medical volunteers and a marine crew, but it also carried teams of young people armed with passion for Jesus to bring the gospel to the Papua New Guinean people. They were welcomed with open arms. Crowds of people gathered to watch their evangelistic skits, public worship, and testimonies. It brought encouragement to the people to feel seen by foreigners who had come from all over the world to minister to them. Many Papua New Guineans received the good news of the gospel and turned to Christ.

One of these Papua New Guineans met me at the ship. She went by the name of Missionary Christine and was a champion of a woman. As she sat across from me, Black, brawny, and weathered, with a huge smile on her face, I was humbled by this woman's presence. Her wide, calloused bare feet and thick, muscular, scarred calves bore evidence of her missionary mileage. I couldn't help but look at my pale White feet and compare her muscular legs to my hairy White ones whose only sacrifice seemed to be the lack of a razor. Christine described her missionary work in Papua New Guinea—how she reached her people by walking hundreds of miles into hard-to-reach remote villages. Her stories were filled with unbelievable hardships of physical endurance laced with miraculous encounters with Jesus. She sat across from me with a smile, wide-eyed, with rapt engagement.

After shared niceties and social exchanges, we finally came to a lull in the conversation, and I realized there was another reason Missionary Christine had come to see me. She came to ask for help. "Sister Rhonda," she began softly, "we are so happy that your organization is sending us teams to share the gospel. But would you tell them that we know that now. Please ask them to send us people to teach us skills so we can have jobs and provide for our families. This is what we really need."

Often seeking higher education is viewed as inferior to "following Jesus" in the sphere of ministry such as Bible teaching, evangelism, and church building, but I am of a different opinion. I believe the church needs a new mission statement more like Captain Kirk's in *Star Trek*: "to explore strange new worlds, to seek out new life, and new civilizations, to boldly go where no one has gone before." This will require hard work, study, and sacrifice. Being qualified for the kingdom is important. Most often, God does call the qualified. Educational and experiential qualifications are necessary if we want to build the kingdom of God.

On the day Jesus called me to be a nurse practitioner, I was working in a rural community as a registered nurse, and on that particular day the physician called out sick. A young couple on their honeymoon came into the clinic. The new wife was in a lot of pain from a urinary tract infection. I was able to collect the urine and use a dip stick that showed her urine contained blood and leukocytes (white blood cells), which definitely indicated that she had an infection. But I couldn't treat her with any medication because that would be out of my scope of practice. Instead, I had to send this young couple an hour away to be seen elsewhere for treatment. I went home that day frustrated and started researching nurse practitioner programs. I felt God wanted me to expand my scope so I could meet the needs of the people who came to me as a healthcare professional.

I had always felt hindered and held back by a medical model that created a bottleneck for access to medical care. Following my first nursing degree and then my bachelor's degree, it was time for me to pursue even higher education so I could help even more people. I remember the intense study, the stress, and the sacrifice to climb the learning curve required to be excellent at what I do. Those years of study required a chunk of my time and attention but also opened the door for me as a medical missionary so that I was able to help people in developing nations and also be registered as a licensed healthcare professional in their country.

As Rick and I got ready to embark on the medical ship, groups of excited young people full of love and passion for Jesus boarded. They would experience life-changing, paradigm-shifting discipleship training. Some of these students were planning on careers in nursing or medicine. Over the course of our time together on the ship, I'd frequently hear students make decisions to leave university to become "missionaries." For them, going into missions and serving God was more important than going back to university. University was sucking the life out of them. Real life was found in the meaningful community they'd formed together during the outreach's intense spiritual environment. That's how they saw it.

As one of the medical professionals on the ship, I had several counseling sessions with students feeling called to missions in a medical capacity. I advised them to return to their studies so they could get the necessary skills to be fully equipped as a missionary serving in a medical ministry.

On another occasion I spoke with a young man who was working with me as a medical volunteer. He was a young, inexperienced emergency medical technician (EMT). Due to the nature of this remote ministry, he was able to participate with skill development that took him beyond his normal scope of practice, performing tasks that he would not be licensed to do in his own country. He obviously loved medicine and had a call on his life to work in this sphere.

I encouraged him to go back to his country to pursue a career in medicine. I explained that if he got licensed, he would be better able to influence the sphere of medicine in the kingdom of God. He responded that he didn't like school and asked why he should pursue years of further education when he could do the things that he was already doing in developing nations. While I recognized this young man's passion for healthcare, I was concerned about proper licensing and ensuring that the people we minister to in developing nations are given our best. If we are not licensed to do skills in our own countries, then we should not be doing them in someone else's.

I see so many Christian young people passionate about Jesus in the areas specific to ministry as a pastor, a missionary, or a Bible teacher, but the percentage who gravitate to academia are few. There are several spheres within the kingdom of God, and we need people to commit to doing whatever it takes to become highly skilled so that God's kingdom can advance in every arena. We need Christians in medical science and research. Who will commit to study and develop skills in these fields?

God wants to give revelation, remedies for healing, and advance the scientific world. There are cures for sickness yet to be discovered. One of my friends has a PhD in marine biology. He said recently, "I've heard groups of Christians say, 'We should pray for a cure for cancer!' but if God gave them the cure for cancer, they wouldn't understand it because they don't have the necessary educational foundation to receive it." Education is undeniably important, but we need to achieve it the correct way.

THE RIGHT RESEARCH

Healthcare providers are encountering a new wave of patients. Patients who come armed with research to let the provider know their diagnosis, to ask for the lab tests they feel they need, and to let us know the alternative treatments or supplements they are taking. I am not threatened by this at all; in fact, there have been times when it's been helpful for me as a nurse practitioner to really listen to the patient. However, "doing your own research" requires an educational foundation that is not as easy as reading a paragraph on a social media platform.

A lack of an understanding of research in medicine can be dangerous. People make misinformed decisions, place themselves at risk, delay treatment, and become susceptible to misinformation. Misinformation can lead to wrong conclusions. It's like the joke about statistics that states that 95 percent of people in prison eat bread; therefore, eating bread leads to a life in prison. Foundational scientific principles for the health of populations are eroding, and I find myself encountering patients who are refusing good, proven treatments because of something they've read or a religious belief about healing. I always respect my patients' rights to their opinion, but that does not stop me from sharing medical research based on evidence and reviewed by highly skilled peers in the field. Being susceptible to misinformation is found in a lack of scientific literacy.

Being scientifically literate means many things, but I feel the main foundations are

1. an understanding of fundamental sciences such as biology, chemistry, and physics;
2. an understanding of statistics, data interpretation, and scientific methods; and
3. an ability to thinking critically (thinking about your thinking so that you think better).

I have a close Christian friend who is a scientist. She is brilliant. Science comes easy to her. She reads research articles for the sheer joy of it. I have called her at times to ask her to look over a study just to make sure I was making a good medical decision, but even my scientist friend will say there is bias and corruption in the research world. Scientists feel pressured to come up with publications so they can get funding, they feel pressure to perform, and they fall in love with their subject and favor positive results, which leads to an incomplete view of the truth. People are people, and as much as educated, academic people can be corrupted, so can eager novices who are influenced by social media and other easily found information online and say, "I've done my own research." If an experienced scientist can be misled by their own bias, then how much more can an individual without a foundation of scientific literacy.

People become susceptible to claims on social media that are amplified by algorithms feeding personal biases. Personal stories and testimonies are more appealing than difficult-to-understand academic studies. Simplified and sensational explanations for complex topics are appealing to all of us. Information overload makes it challenging to understand credible resources, and if one has any distrust of authority, government, or pharmaceutical companies, it increases susceptibility to error. Medical science and research are good, but Jesus must be kept at the center.

Another friend who has a doctorate told me a story about his brother who is a scientist involved in cutting-edge medical research related to one of the world's leading concerns in global health. Both my friend and his brother have brilliant minds, and both pursued professions in the academic world of science. Their father was a missionary for most of his life, yet he strongly encouraged his sons to pursue higher education. My friend told me that his brother was frustrated with his research and was repeatedly hitting a wall in his struggle for a medical breakthrough for a global health concern. Countless grueling, rigorous hours of defeat and failure resulted in discouragement and scientific fatigue.

While he poured out his heart to his family, his father jumped into the conversation. His missionary father did not have the academic, educational background of his sons, but he suggested they pray and ask God for wisdom. After some prayer, the missionary dad felt he heard God speak to him and suggested his son try what he had heard in prayer. His son looked at him incredulously, reminded him that he wasn't a scientist, and let him know that he had tried everything already. The brother returned home and went back to grinding out his experiments, but he could not get the words of his father out of his mind. In a last-ditch effort, he changed the way he performed the experiment, implemented the idea his father had suggested, and came up with the answer. His research became a key solution for a global crisis that causes one of the leading diseases in the world today.

The son had the necessary educational foundation, and God used the missionary dad to drop the key to the breakthrough. The answer came through years of study, training, and scientific research, with some final tweaking by Jesus. As healthcare professionals we need both. We need our educational foundation and all the medical knowledge available around us while we sit beside Jesus at the center.

CHAPTER 7
WHAT IS GOOD HEALTH?

Nacho: "I'm not listening to you! You only believe in science. That's probably why we never win!"

Esquelito: "We never win because you are fat!"

NACHO LIBRE

In 2017 I completed some missionary training in a tropical location. The training center was located on the main street of the town where tourists came by to enjoy the ocean view. Many local vendors set up stalls in hopes to sell their crafts to the strolling tourists. The vendors' location also put them along the path of eager, young missionary students leaving classes every day.

One day I stopped by a local vendor selling her artwork. We started talking, and I asked about her life and her spiritual beliefs. She shared her frustration with the daily stream of passionate young people exiting the missionary school. They walked past her small sales booth and never bought anything from her. "But," she complained, "they always try to save my soul." I certainly understood how this could get tiresome for her.

As I listened with an empathetic ear, the woman poured out a flood of hurtful and frustrating examples of encounters with the Christian young people. She told me about her friend whose hair never grew. Her friend was bald, but other than that she was healthy and lived life to the fullest. Whenever students from the school saw her friend, they assumed she had cancer and was undergoing chemotherapy treatments. They would gather around her to pray for healing from something she didn't have. The roadside vendor felt this was insensitive, and as she told me the story I couldn't help but roll my eyes in frustration and agree with her. There was no relational equity built with the receiver of prayer, there were no questions asked, there was no time taken to hear her story. The inexperienced students looked at the outward appearance and were led to the wrong conclusion.

To be honest, we do this a lot in medicine. We make assumptions about the people we see and often come to the wrong conclusions about their needs or the status of their health. When my patients schedule an appointment with me, the receptionist asks, "What is the main reason for your visit?" The patient's answer is logged as the chief complaint and becomes the basis of a clinical encounter with a sick patient. I look through my list and know immediately which visits will be quick and which will require more time. There are chief complaints that cause us to groan inwardly; ones that make us suspicious; and ones that make our hearts beat a little faster, intrigue us, or even make us roll our eyes. Our job is based on identifying problems, and people come to us as the problem-solvers. But good health is more than fixing problems.

What does it mean to be healthy? What does healing really look like? Can someone in a wheelchair be healthy? Can someone who looks successful and physically healthy on the outside be sick on the inside?

The World Health Organization (WHO) gave a definition for health in 1948: "Health is a state of complete physical, mental, and social well-being and not merely the absence of disease or infirmity."[1] In 1986, my first year of nursing, WHO decided the definition needed an addendum and added: "Health is a resource for everyday life, not the objective of living. It is a positive concept emphasizing social and personal resources as well as physical capacities."[2] This definition is extremely important because it tells us that good health is wholistic, it is a resource for a good life, and it is not as simple as being free of disease or infirmity.

Over the years, I have worked in community health and development both nationally and internationally. One of the best illustrations for teaching about good health is a lesson available through Community Health Evangelism (CHE) titled "What Is Good Health?" I have used CHE to teach in developing nations; I also frequently use this lesson in my practice, as it helps both my patients and colleagues to understand what it means to be healthy. The lesson begins with the story of Mr. Mafu:

Mr. Mafu had a very nice horse. As he rode to work one day, the horse stepped into a hole. Mr. Mafu fell off and broke his leg. His neighbor, a good friend, took him home and the family called the traditional doctor.

The doctor told Mr. Mafu the neighbor had brought this evil on him. He also advised Mr. Mafu to go to the hospital where his leg was put into a cast. While he stayed in the hospital, Mr. Mafu kept saying, "It shows you cannot even trust your best friend!"

When the cast came off, Mr. Mafu was so glad the leg was healed, but he wanted to go and pay back the evil his friend had done. From that day he started to do wrong things against his neighbor.[3]

This tragic and silly story ends with a question for the group of listeners. I've asked the same question to my patients many times: "Is Mr. Mafu healthy?"

They always give the same answer: "No, he's not healthy because he is filled with anger and is going to go and hurt his neighbor."

I respond with the same comment: "But his broken leg is fixed!"

They invariably push back, "Yes, but he's angry!"

This is why the WHO definition of good health is so important. Good health is not merely the absence of disease or infirmity. If we look solely at outside appearances, we can make assumptions about what needs to be healed based on the medical problems listed on the patient's chart. If only good health were that simple. Appearances aren't always accurate, as we saw with the students praying over a vibrant, healthy woman whose "ailment" amounted simply to being born with alopecia.

Once I've made the point about good health being more than a healed body, I take the CHE training to the next steps. The first chapter of Genesis best describes *shalom*, the concept of peace, well-being, and completeness. When God created us, he made us whole complete beings living in harmony with him, with ourselves, with our environment, and with others. Adam and Eve chose fruit that led to death, and it fractured this harmony. We live with the evidence of that decision today. Can we be healthy? Can *shalom* be restored?

When I ask patients what they think it means to be healthy, I draw an illustration to help them visualize God's full design for the role harmony plays in our health. I have used the exam table paper to draw a circle and divide it into four sections. Good health can be broken into four quadrants that require deeper understanding and assessment to find the root cause of illness. Good health means I am in harmony with myself, with others, with my environment, and with God.

Good health means being in harmony with:

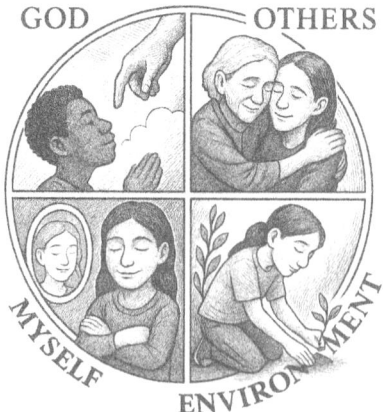

This simple tool has helped bring incredible insight into the lives of my patients. I have seen patients come into my examination room with abdominal pain only to realize their real problem was unforgiveness.

Now, pretend you're in my examination room and I've just drawn a big circle on the paper lining the table and divided the circle into fourths. Let's look at the first quadrant.

HARMONY WITH MYSELF

What does it mean to be in "harmony with myself"? I have asked my patients this question and I'm always amazed at their answers. Many of us do not know the answer. Especially if we have been raised in a religion or culture that feels it is honorable to put ourselves last, the concept of "harmony with myself" can make us uncomfortable. It can feel like we are aligning with worldly philosophy, selfishness, or even narcissism.

Several years ago, before I became a nurse practitioner, I worked at a small clinic in rural New Brunswick, Canada. I was a community health nurse, mostly involved in project development aimed at needs within the community. I felt burned out running all of these programs and I didn't seem to see any improvements. I needed more training in the area of fixing the problems in the community and decided to attend a community development conference in Toronto, Ontario, Canada.

I met one of the conference speakers, a seasoned therapist who was teaching the practice of mindfulness. He was Jewish but he attributed more success with achieving harmony in his life to Buddhism. We talked about our personal challenges and beliefs, and he listened with great interest to my stories of my current community work, my missionary work in Haiti, my acts of service to my community, and my busy family life.

After getting to know several details about my life, he made a startling comment: "Rhonda, if you loved yourself more, you would be a better Christian."

There are moments in life when a sentence or a phrase from

someone else can seem like a spiritual slap—this was one of them. I felt immediate opposition and irritation. My outer response to him remained silent, but I was shouting on the inside, "Who do you think you are? You're a Buddhist saying that to me? I am a Christian. I am the one who has the truth!"

I walked away in turmoil, stumbling over his statement, conflicting thoughts and emotions swirling. I was embarrassed that he saw through my selfless, sacrificial service that others seemed to admire, and I felt shame that my Christian example was obviously not thrilling for him. A rush of memorized Bible verses about dying to myself daily blasted on a self-justifying megaphone in my brain. But during it all I heard God's still, small voice: "Rhonda, you need to love your neighbor as yourself."

I quickly answered, "God, you know I love my neighbor. I have constantly laid down my life for others. You've seen my missionary life. You know how I've made sacrifices for others. I've given away all I have. I've gone to places you've asked me to!"

His answer came in two words: "As yourself."

As we began to have a quiet conversation, the megaphone stopped and the emotions settled.

"As yourself."

I thought about the passage where Jesus informed his disciples of the two most important commandments:

Jesus replied, "The most important commandment is this: Listen, O Israel! The LORD our God is the one and only LORD. And you must love the LORD your God with all your heart, all your soul, all your mind, and all your strength. The second is equally important: 'Love your neighbor as yourself.' No other commandment is greater than these." (Mark 12:29–31 NLT)

I kept hearing the words "as yourself" repeated over and over.

The answer began to take shape in my heart. It was not an easy one, and it also confirmed that my Buddhist friend was right. If I am loving my neighbor as myself, then the way I love myself will be the level with which I love my neighbor. This was a difficult concept for me. I had been taught to deny myself, to die to myself, to carry my cross daily.

While these Scriptures did battle in my head, a memory flashed in my mind. I was twenty-two years old, so excited about the newfound freedom I had discovered as a new Christian. I was discussing the book of Romans with a friend, quoting verses about dying to my old ways, my old self. Maybe he thought I needed further counsel. "I would agree we need to die to self," he said, "but it seems to me there are a whole lot of people stuck in the dying part and not walking out the resurrected part. What about living, Rhonda?"

I returned to the conversation about loving myself that God had started with me. I asked God another question: "God, if I am not loving myself, then what have I been doing for other people? Haven't I loved all the people I have served all these years as a missionary?"

I didn't get any answer. He just let me think about it. God is good that way. He is not harsh or unkind. He lets us come to conclusions that may be hurtful, without a voice of condemnation. He is a heavenly Father who sits with us as we come to conclusions. He waits patiently with hugs when realization hits.

And it hit. The realization that all my love for others wasn't love at all. Years of self-denial, service, and self-sacrifice were based on my own neediness. A personal need for validation to make me feel good about me—the person I put last every day. If Jesus loves me, then shouldn't I love me?

Being in harmony with myself begins by loving myself. It also means that I should know myself. I should be in a continual place of self-discovery. We often tend to think we know ourselves, but our need for connection can supersede our identity. Rather than focus on our own personal giftings, desires, dreams, and visions, we conform to the expectations of others so we feel acceptance. It takes courage to know who we are.

As a nurse practitioner running a family practice, I have developed an expertise in treating mental health. I think this is mainly due to having lived with anxiety and depression for several years. I learned to manage my anxiety with lifestyle strategies that helped me to navigate life despite fear and constant exhausting mental rumination. Years of personal growth, inner healing, and professional experience have helped me to develop an expertise. My personal struggles have made me very empathetic and given me insight into the mental health of my patients.

Since the onset of genetic testing, we now have access to personal genetic information that can help us understand our unique mental processes. Understanding ourselves helps us to work with our weaknesses and makes us more self-forgiving. In recent years I sent my DNA to a genetic testing lab to explore risk factors for disease and possible impaired processes around cognitive function. My results identified at least three neurotransmitter receptor mutations that affected suboptimal serotonin and dopamine production and utilization. These mutations are associated with addictions, ADHD, and other mental health disorders. The literature also noted that these conditions are exacerbated when factors such as childhood trauma have occurred. This discovery opened a moment of understanding for me and an opportunity for self-forgiveness. My childhood trauma surrounding my little brother's near-death experience had haunted me secretly for years, inhibiting true harmony with myself.

Another requirement to being in harmony with myself means I care for my body that God created. I look at it in the mirror and thank God for my body. I feed it well, I make sure it doesn't get too heavy or too thin, I make sure it gets proper sleep, and I exercise it and treat it well.

During our Discipleship Training School with YWAM, Rick and I spent two months on a small group of islands in the Pacific. The people group of these islands had the highest rates of diabetes and tuberculosis in the world. I met a pastor who had been serving there for several years and listened to his frustration with the poor access to food, the alarming rates of diabetes among the people, and the lack of education surrounding nutrition in these islands. While venting his frustration, he blurted out, "The devil is killing these people with diabetes!"

I agree the Enemy can both directly and indirectly kill, steal, and destroy people. I also know that if we lack understanding and live in ignorance about our physical health, it can lead to poor health and even an early death. Living in a geographical location that has poor access to proper nutrition will lead to poor health. Choosing to abuse our body by not feeding it properly, not maintaining it by preventive practices, and not running the engine through regular exercise can lead to illness.

I have personally witnessed healing meetings where people are praying for the healing of type 2 diabetes or heart disease while it's completely evident the individual's lifestyle was a contributing factor to their chronic disease. These prayers may be a little late in the game. Why does the person receiving prayer have heart disease or diabetes? Did they lack education? Do they have diabetes because of emotional eating associated with loneliness or trauma? Do they have heart disease due to stress and worry because they needed to perform for approval? God can still heal current issues, but if we don't experience healing for root causes and address these issues, we will continue to experience poor health.

For the river of healing to flow in harmony within us, we need to consider how we might be obstructing the flow by our own choices. Thankfully, the Holy Spirit is with us and will help us identify necessary steps for us to take so we can regain inner harmony.

Let's move onto the second quadrant, harmony with others, to help us better understand good health.

HARMONY WITH OTHERS

What does it mean to be in harmony with others? Do I have friends? Do I have community around me? What about my relationship with my family? Am I living in peace with my neighbors?

We discussed the story of Mr. Mafu and his determination to seek vengeance on his neighbor, and we agreed he was not healthy. Anger, unresolved conflicts, and unforgiveness are all like slivers in our skin. The body's immune system responds to the foreign body by causing inflammation at the site. It creates pus around the sliver to isolate it and keep it from affecting the rest of the body but also creates pressure that will naturally push the object out through the skin. Sometimes if the sliver is too deep, people need professional help to remove it.

Issues in our physical brains can also keep us from harmony with others. Dopamine and serotonin are such important neurotransmitters and are linked to feelings of positive experiences in social settings, feelings of closeness, trust, and satisfaction within relationships. For those of us operating with lower levels of these important neurotransmitters, sadness, lack of motivation, social anxiety, and addictions are struggles that are real. I have several patients who suffer the effects of trauma, abuse, abandonment, and the list goes on. We live in a broken world. Being in harmony with others is likely the most challenging aspect of our health to overcome because of the trauma and broken trust that was inflicted on us by others.

One of my patients listened intently regarding the need to be in harmony with others. She was struggling with homelessness, maintaining employment, and severe anxiety and depression. I started her on medication and had her come back the following week.

At the follow-up visit she wanted to share her thoughts after we discussed being in harmony with others. "When I left your office, I walked out to the road and sat on the curb to think. I realized I had unforgiveness in my heart toward my mother, so I forgave her, and I felt something inside of me shift." Over the next few months, I was able to witness the power of forgiveness walked out in this young woman's life.

Isolationism is extremely unhealthy. I have patients who justify social isolation by claiming to be introverts. An introverted personality simply reflects a preference for less stimulating environments, a need for deeper conversations with others, and a need for times of solitude to feel balanced and energized. Withdrawing from community under the guise of introversion can be rooted in an unhealthy isolationism associated with social anxiety and rooted in a fear of rejection. I often see addiction attached to social isolation. Alcohol or drugs work well as neurotransmitter blockers to decrease anxiety. They create a short-term sense of peace and give boldness to engage with others. Although these substances appear to work well, they are a short-term fix that carry a bundle of unhealthy outcomes without dealing with the root cause of anxiety.

We are meant to be together. We are created for community, and we grow emotionally healthy when we live and walk together with others. However, many individuals suffer from a poverty spirit and an orphan spirit. These two seem to go hand in hand and keep us from receiving love. A poverty spirit keeps us from recognizing our value, and an orphan spirit makes us feel like we don't belong. These two cosmic spirits keep many people isolated. They often accomplish this by disguising themselves as part of a person's personality.

I come from a long line of hermits who identify as introverts. This doesn't mean they don't have close family members they can feel comfortable with, but it does mean that circles outside of this inner group are limited. There is also a lengthy history of alcoholism and loneliness in my family, especially on my maternal side. Even as a child I experienced a lot of social anxiety and shyness. As a young girl I played independently and had only a few close friends. This followed me into my teenage years.

To feel courage and acceptance with others, I smoked cannabis every lunch hour, smoked cigarettes, and on weekends drank an over-abundance of alcohol. I constantly acted out with high-risk, impulsive behavior like racing and jumping cars, motorbikes, and even horses. I was a teacher's nightmare. I almost didn't graduate from high school, developed an eating disorder, and then developed a shopping craze for clothing during college that turned into credit card debt to support my lifestyle. During that time, I had very few close relationships but was popular on a superficial level.

Around age twenty-two, I turned my life over to Jesus and things turned around, but this didn't put a complete end to the social anxiety in my life; many of the behaviors simply adapted to Christian culture. Life in a Christian community does not insulate us from painful and hurtful experiences with others. In fact, the hurt we experience in a

Christian community can be more painful than in a secular setting because it affects us at the deepest levels of trust.

When we are loved, we feel valuable and have a deep sense of belonging, but when we do not feel worthy of love or are skeptical of relationships, we pull back into social isolation. Social isolation results in social anxiety that is usually rooted in a fear of rejection. It is impossible to have harmony with others when we pull back into fear. Fear isolates us, has negative effects on our mental health, and can lead to depression, anxiety, and cognitive decline. The highest risk of suicide is male middle- or older-age men who are experiencing social isolation.

Once I had gained harmony with myself through dealing with my childhood trauma, I was able to understand the critical nature of harmony with others, so I began to work on my relationships. After ten-hour days in my family practice, I turned away the tendency to demand my time to myself. I said yes to holding a small group in my house weekly. On my one day off I booked coffee dates with anyone who wanted to meet with me. I joined a ladies' Bible study once weekly. I'll be honest, this community-building exercise was exhausting, but I kept pushing against the tendency to be suspicious of people, to want to isolate, and I worked at pushing aside any fear of rejection.

For two years my home was full of people two to three nights a week. My day off became booked with social engagements, and I even joined a ministry at my local church. I began to sense a change in my relationship with others. I developed a large community and tribe of people, the fear of rejection began to disappear, and my sense of loneliness was turned into a healthy sense of acceptance among friends. Building community required work. The very thing I had tried to avoid was the answer to bringing harmony with others to my life.

Building community, making friends, and fostering friendship creates a life of harmony with others and this leads to good health.

The third quadrant, harmony with our environment, is another area to explore for the root cause of illness.

HARMONY WITH OUR ENVIRONMENT

During my nine months on the medical ship in Papua New Guinea, I often encountered illnesses associated with the environment. During a busy clinic day, a tall, quiet father and his four children waited in line to be seen. When isolated tribal communities heard the medical ship was coming, word spread to remote communities located farther inland. People walked or paddled for days to meet the ship. The local Papua New Guinean health center worker informed me the father had paddled for three days from a community upriver.

He registered his family and stood in front of me, gently pushing his four shy, young children from behind his legs to be examined. He wanted to make sure they were up to date with their childhood immunizations. As he presented each child to me, he looked on proudly with a huge smile. He likely had big dreams for these beautiful children. He appeared to be a proud, good father, like any father I would see in my own country.

The first child he pushed forward was a wide-eyed six-year-old boy. I did my usual assessment and noticed his enlarged belly, which I often associated with parasites. I expected to treat the boy with antiparasitic medication, but as I pressed my fingers over his abdomen I felt a huge mass. It started on his left upper quadrant and extended completely across his left lower abdomen. I traced the edges of this mass to his lower right quadrant. This thing was huge. I palpated the edges of this huge mass, which didn't appear to cause him pain while I prodded his abdomen, in disbelief. I had never encountered anything like this in my years of practice.

Thankfully, locally trained Papua New Guinean physicians, highly experienced in the area's common diseases, accompanied us on the ship's medical outreaches. Foreign-trained medical professionals were often stumped by the specific conditions encountered there. I searched in desperation for Dr. Mana, a highly trained local doctor who specialized in tropical medicine. When I found him, I pulled the doctor away from the line of patients in front of him and breathlessly babbled off my findings with an urgent request for him to see this child.

He walked over and began to palpate the child's swollen belly. "Oh? You haven't seen this before?" I listened, wide-eyed, while he calmly explained, "The mass you are feeling is his spleen. His spleen has enlarged from chronic malaria. This is called hyper-reactive malarial splenomegaly syndrome, or HMSS."

I looked at the child, wondering about the treatment and the prognosis. How could I fix this? Was this treatable? I asked Dr. Mana what could be done.

"Well, you can treat him with malaria medication for a lengthy period, but this won't change if he keeps getting malaria."

One by one I assessed this kind father's beautiful children, and one by one I continued to be astonished by the size of each child's spleen. I thought about his three-day paddle to get to me. Medication would only last for a short period, until the malaria-ridden environment exacerbated their condition. I stood there helpless in front of the smiling father and four children who found their way back behind his legs.

The local nurse walked over to me. With a sigh, she said, "Yes, this family lives way upriver where there are many swamps. We heard that the healthcare workers have been reporting these cases to the Department of Health, and there are plans to move this village somewhere else."

I was grateful for her words. It offered me some hope. Before I sent them off with medication and mosquito nets, I watched the father nod and eagerly listen to the local community worker as she gave him some preventive education and discussed how to take the medication. I laid my hand on each child and prayed for healing.

I know God heals. I believed he could shrink down these spleens easily and this would be a miracle, but this did not happen when I prayed for these children. Healing would require God-given wisdom of medical science, public health guidelines, and government assistance to move this family to a safer setting. Healing for this family would come once they were living in harmony with their environment.

I mentioned earlier the people group in the Pacific with high diabetes rates. Other issues existed in this community that were far more complicated. This people group lived in a geographical location that had been used for nuclear testing, and they had high cancer rates. The land was facing rising sea levels that were causing land erosion and poor soil content, contributing to food insecurity. In addition, overcrowding and decreased available housing led to multiple problems: increased rates of TB, and homes that held multiple people often sleeping together in shifts, contributing to unsafe personal spaces for young girls and teenage pregnancy. These issues can all be traced back to the fractured disharmony with the environment. Until that is stabilized, good health and healing will constantly be hindered for these unfortunate people.

Some of us may need to change our environments if we are to be healthy. A variety of patients in my practice endure complex environmental problems that contribute to their illnesses. The source of these issues cannot be discovered in a fifteen-minute office visit. It takes adequate time to build relationships with patients for this type of information to emerge.

On one occasion I was praying for healing over one of my patients regarding a physical illness. I heard God say, "His problem is foundational." I asked God what he meant. He said, "He needs a home and a stable living environment."

I questioned the patient about his living environment and confirmed what I'd heard God say in my spirit. The man lacked housing and was living in his car. He had been living in a geographical location with some of the highest rents in the country, combined with a housing crisis in an area with no affordable housing.

My prescription for this patient's healing was not a drug, it was not surgery, and it was not a medical procedure. I recommended he move to another state and community with affordable housing and more stability.

This surprised my patient. He told me he felt called to this community by God. He was staying, despite the difficulties he faced in his environment.

When a patient tells me that God told them something different from what I feel I am hearing from the Holy Spirit, it's game over. I sat back and gave him some medicine for his present issue, but I knew his health would continue to deteriorate unless his environment improved.

A week later this patient returned to my office for follow up. He told me he had prayed about what we'd discussed. He thanked me for my words and shared that a friend called to invite him to join a ministry in another state, and he felt God releasing him from his present commitment. He moved to a better environment with stable housing, more ministry, and better employment options. His health could improve now that he was in harmony with his environment.

Being in harmony with our environment is all about where we work, the house we live in, and the geographical location where we live. Do we have a place to live that is stable? Are the walls painted with lead paint? Do we live next to a petroleum plant? What about the possibility of floods, of earthquakes, of volcanoes? Is our neighborhood a safe one or are there gangs and high crime rates? Do we work in a stressful, toxic work environment?

This is an important checkpoint for each of us to ask ourselves: Am I living in harmony with my environment? If my environment is not safe, if my workplace is volatile, if the air is polluted, if my housing is not stable, then I am not in harmony with my environment and I will be unhealthy. This eventually works into my emotional and physical health.

I have spent most of my life in ministry serving as a missionary in medical missions. A lifestyle in missions often means moving from place to place, and although this can be adventurous and rewarding, it can also result in an inability to create harmony with our environment. When our environment is changing frequently, it destabilizes the mind. Instability leads to anxiety.

I often see clients in my practice with physical illnesses that I know are linked to the patient's disharmony with their environment. Everyone needs a familiar safe space. Constant change can impair cognition, especially as we get older.

I realize we can't always control everything in our environment, but we can make choices to bring as much harmony with our environment as possible. Our health depends upon it.

As we approach the fourth quadrant, we can see how harmony with God affects us in every area of our lives.

HARMONY WITH GOD

A few years ago, I went walking alone by the beach close to where I live in Hawaii. I felt in my heart that I lacked love. I didn't feel like I loved God the way he deserved to be loved. How could I ever be thankful enough, grateful enough, loving enough to God to be in perfect harmony with him?

I turned my eyes upward and said, "God, I don't feel like I love you the way you should be loved."

He quickly answered, "Rhonda, that's because I need to love you into loving me."

I thought of the verse about how we love him because he first loved us (1 John 4:9). Love must first come from God. It is not something we can generate from ourselves. It all comes down to the simple act of receiving his love. If we can't allow ourselves to be loved, we will not be able to love ourselves or others.

I stood on the beach, arms wide open. "Okay, God, come and love me and I will receive your love. Go ahead and love me."

I didn't feel anything physical or spiritual, but I had given God permission. That was all he required. Receiving the love of God is the single most important form of healing I have ever experienced.

For so many of us, we keep a distance, however intentional, from God. His standards are so holy, his calling to obedience so intense. Our natural human response to such high expectations is fear. Ironically, the number one answer to overcoming fear is the love of God. Receiving the love of God drives out fear. The Bible says that perfect love casts out fear (1 John 4:18). As we receive God's love, we experience a personal connection with him unlike any other. It is possible to know, deep in our hearts, that we are loved by him.

John was one of the twelve disciples of Jesus, and it is believed he wrote five books of the Bible. John referred to himself at least five times as the disciple whom Jesus loved. It is a blatant phrase and a confident one: "I am the one he loved." John obviously knew he was loved enough to write it down. During the last supper, John wrote that he reclined, or laid against, Jesus: "Now there was leaning on Jesus' bosom one of his disciples, whom Jesus loved. Simon Peter therefore motioned to him to ask who it was of whom he spoke. . . . Then, leaning back on Jesus' breast, he said to Him, 'Lord who is it?'" (John 13:23–25 NKJV).

There are a couple of things to note in this passage. First, John was openly demonstrative and affectionate with Jesus. He even wrote the details of physically laying his head on the chest of Jesus. Second, John also seems to note that the other disciples were aware he was loved. He describes an occasion where Peter went through John to ask a question because he knew John had favor. Regardless, John knew he was loved. I believe a lot of healing would occur in my patients if they knew they were loved by a loving God. Not until we know we are loved, can we be in harmony with ourselves, with others, with our environment, and with God.

The greatest form of healing for all manner of physical illnesses is not found in medicine or supplements, nutrition or exercise. It is not found in a fire tunnel or a healing line. The greatest form of healing that could solve 95 percent of all illnesses in the Western world would occur if people felt the love of God and lived daily in harmony with him. God's love, indeed, is the basis of good health.

CHAPTER 8

WHEN THE GIFTS OF THE SPIRIT MEET MEDICAL SCIENCE

The good physician treats the disease;
the great physician treats the patient who has the disease.
SIR WILLIAM OSLER

I am no stranger to extreme physical training. I have trained for marathons and long-distance swimming. I have known my share of hard work. But tree planting is another level of physical endurance that weeds out the strong from the weak. I have watched strong grown men fall to the ground in sobs. This is what I discovered when Rick and I managed a silviculture, or tree planting, program in northern Canada. We did this as missionaries for six years in the 1990s.

The program provided employment opportunities and job training for the local community, and every tree planting shift was the same. The groans and complaints began as disheveled planters with aching muscles emerged from warm sleeping bags to cold, damp clothing with wet work boots from the previous days. The cold early morning breakfasts were devoid of joy, mechanically consumed for the purpose of energy, and mindless chewing replaced conversations as planters hurriedly washed down mouthfuls of food with gulps of coffee.

Lunches, water bottles, and backpacks were meticulously prepared for another sixteen-hour day.

The drive from the tree plant base to the plant site was often arduous and intensive. Small wagons hauled the planters through muddy roads, bogs, and difficult-to-reach areas. I'd watch them drive off with the four-wheelers pulling wagons full of planters huddled under tarps to ward off the pouring rain. Sometimes the wagons would hit uneven terrain and tip the entire crew into the swamp.

Planters became so adamant in their competitiveness to plant trees that they would endure the wet, muddy clothes to hit their numbers for the day. Every tree planted represented an accumulation of money; wasted time meant less trees, so physical comfort took a back seat to the motivating power of financial gain. Nothing could stand in their way—until a local family of beavers moved in and threatened access to one of our reforestation areas.

The beaver is symbolic in Canada because of its historical significance in the country's fur trade during the seventh and eighteenth centuries. Beavers are amazing, industrious, hard-working creatures, and although the public finds them cute and admirable, they became a daily frustration to maintaining access to our plant area.

The furry creatures were determined to build a dam on a small brook running parallel to the road that provided access to our tree plant area. The beaver dam held back the water's flow, which then washed out the road, leaving a deep crevice to cross with the four-wheelers and wagons.

It became a competition of wits. In the evening, Rick and a few guys would go and pull the dam apart and try to build up the deep ditch in the road. But the beavers worked the night shift, and by morning the flow of water washed out the road again. Rick would come back every night convinced he had won the battle. "We really pulled it apart this time!" he would say with a look of determination on his tired face. They'd removed the dam, and the small brook flowed freely again.

But every day was the same. The parties would arrive at the location to find the dam was rebuilt through the night, the rebuilt crossing was washed out, and they faced another harrowing ride across the deep crevice. The ride to the plant site became the talk of legends that included speed, skill, and inertia amid the sounds of roaring engines and screams of planters hanging on for dear life.

The battle didn't end until Fish and Wildlife officers came out, trapped the beaver family, and relocated it to an alternative location.

This story is a physical example of a few spiritual lessons. Barriers or impingement can hinder the life-giving water that flows from within us. As professionals in healthcare, do we allow the healing river to dry up on our watch? Can flow be hindered? Can the river be blocked or restricted? Can the forceful flow slow to a trickle?

We can get distracted by dealing with debris and impingements without removing the direct cause. This situation becomes even more complicated when our very profession stands as the dam blocking the flow of the Holy Spirit.

Every day in my clinic, anxious patients look at me with tear-filled eyes, wringing their hands, squirming in their seats, desperately wanting a solution for their illnesses—a solution I may or may not have. What if a solution doesn't come? The answer to this can be challenging, especially since medicine is taking credit for healing when it shouldn't. The medical profession has been given far too much credit for healing. The basis of our profession is to bring healing to the sick. Unfortunately, the television and movie industry has influenced our public image, elevating us to sometimes superhero status. Further credit comes from our accrediting bodies, from academia, and from professional associations. We are a lofty crew.

While the science of medicine is good, medicine does not possess all the solutions for illness or all the answers about healing. Is healing always immediate or can it take a long time? Does healing always occur the same way and through the same process? Does healing always require faith? There is one answer to these questions that is always true: healing is complex. It can be miraculous and instantaneous, or it can take a long time. Healing may occur in an area that we didn't anticipate and may occur with or without faith. The process for healing is not always the same.

BUILT ON SCIENCE

What attracted us to healthcare? The vocation of nursing is a part of who I am. I am called to mercy and called to healing. I think this is the same for all professions surrounding the science of medicine. We want to see people healed, we want to alleviate suffering, and we want to see people healthy. Our medical professions are built on science, which is built on four key principles:

1. Empiricism: Trust what you can see and measure.
2. Parsimony: The simplest explanation is most likely the correct one.
3. Replicability: Others should get the same results if they do the same thing.
4. Falsifiability: There should be a way to test it and show that it is false if it really is.

The scientific method is incredibly exciting, and as I said earlier, it is something I have consistently been drawn to, because I always want the best for my patients. I can get lost in research studies before I finally conclude on a certain medicine or a procedure. People deserve the best treatment, and I love it when a plan works. I can't tell you the dopamine rush that comes from a plan of care that lands on one medication that treats three different problems. This likely sounds quite boring to most, but for those of us in medicine the thrill is real. I love how the scientific method is unapologetic, rigid, sniffs out error, takes authority, and gives confidence to the user.

Science exposes snake oil and rescues vulnerable people from being manipulated and deceived. The apostle Paul talks about being careful with snake oil when he says, "Have nothing to do with godless myths and old wives' tales" (1 Timothy 4:7 NIV). What does the term *old wives' tales* mean? The phrase originates from earlier days when older married women were traditional keepers of domestic knowledge and medical advice. Much of this advice was not based on scientific evidence, and over the years as medical research developed, many tales proved inaccurate and even harmful. The biblical reference in 1 Timothy encourages wisdom and discernment around what we accept as truth and what we allow to influence our life.

What does it mean to be a Christian medical professional? It means we have Jesus Christ living in us. We work in partnership with the Holy Spirit, who gives us supernatural gifts for the purpose of building the body of Christ and the kingdom of God. As Jesus promised when he ascended to his Father, he sent the Holy Spirit in his place. The Holy Spirit comes bearing gifts. Some of these gifts are air-dropped on the spot and some come by special request. At the same time, we have an education based in medical science. We pull from two very different worlds—like oil and vinegar that need to be shaken together before being poured out.

Many of us have not managed to bring the two together, but this book is written to tell you that it is possible to be an excellent health-care professional with a foundation of good scientific knowledge while walking in our spiritual gifts. We sharpen our clinical skills through practice, and we learn to sharpen our spiritual gifts through practice. Just like we physically build muscle in our bodies, the gifts from the Holy Spirit must be stirred up, exercised, and practiced so the spiritual muscle enlarges and strengthens.

Science must be a foundational pillar in my practice as a nurse practitioner, but if I solely depend on science, I exclude God completely from my practice. Prayers become the last-ditch effort for healing and a feel-good roll of the dice into the universe. My prayers for patients become wishful thinking and go no higher than the ceiling, and I will make all kinds of assumptions about the will and character of God. Science is good, but why did Jesus tell us to pray? The answer is simple: prayer makes a difference.

Jesus always prayed to his Father for insight. He said that everything he did was based on his ongoing present communication with his Father in heaven and he wouldn't do anything if his Father did not give him guidance first. Jesus explains this in his own words in John 5:19: "The Son can do nothing by himself; he can do only what he sees the Father doing, because whatever the Father does the Son does also" (NIV).

Since this is the case for Jesus, then it is the same for us. If I depend on something that worked in the past, I am not participating in the present. We cannot take a spiritual methodology that may have worked elsewhere and create cookie-cutter methods that we heard worked well in another ministry setting and expect the same result every time. Jesus may have a fresh piece of advice, a new remedy, or a prophetic insight for the individual in front of me who needs healing. It comes down to a combination of applying what we know for the patient and depending on Jesus. We do not try to make medical science spiritual, and the reverse is true as well; we don't try to make spiritual gifts fit into the scientific method.

KNOWING HIS VOICE

My husband and I have been married for thirty-seven years. Sometimes one of us will make a comment to the other and laugh. The two of us understand what it means because of an experience we shared, and it becomes an inside joke. It is the same with Jesus.

He often will minister to us in ways that we understand and speak in ways that are personal and meaningful. It can be so personal that sometimes we think it must be our own thoughts, but as we grow closer to Jesus and learn to hear his voice, we begin to recognize when he is speaking. Jesus said, "My sheep hear my voice" (John 10:27), and his voice can change everything. He does not speak to us all in the same language. I am not talking about languages like English or French. He knows what we know and understands how we think. Often Jesus will quote to me a movie line that he knows I find funny or a lyric from a song on the radio that was meaningful to me at a difficult time. It is something that only the two of us share.

One time in ministry I was incredibly discouraged. I seemed invisible and unheard to those around me. Alone in my office, I climbed under my desk and curled myself into a ball while pulling in my office chair behind me. If anyone walked into my office, they wouldn't see this grown woman in a fetal position under her desk. At least I could have a good cry in privacy. In that dark moment, a movie scene flashed on the screen of my imagination. It was the scene from the movie *The Help* when Aibileen says to the little girl, Mae Mobley, "You is kind, you is smart, you is important." Jesus knew I had watched this movie, and this simple line from a movie lifted me from discouragement to joy.

When I asked Jesus about the way he speaks to me, he said, "Rhonda, when I speak to you, I speak 'Rhonda.'" He speaks to me in a way I will get.

Throughout my day I hear him speak to me. He reminds me of a lab test I should have ordered. He whispers a diagnosis in my ear that I may not have thought of. He reminds me of another patient with similar symptoms so I can come to a better conclusion. He even checks me if I make a mistake on an order or a medication. I can't imagine doing this without his presence.

It didn't always used to be this way. I have been involved with taking care of the sick for nearly four decades. Partnering with Jesus in my profession has been a long journey to understand my identity as a follower of Jesus who opens the flow for the Holy Spirit for healing to those around me. I always longed to see miracles, but my definition of a miracle left me disappointed. Eventually all I had to offer was good godly wisdom, medicine, and my spiritual gift of mercy.

I knew God used me to share his love and mercy to a suffering world, but I felt there was more for me. I didn't push in further to practice my gifts of prophecy or healing because I didn't understand my identity. I had no sense of the spiritual authority that I carried. I longed to believe the words of Jesus about instantaneous healing by the laying on of hands. My longing for the gift of healing was real, but my understanding of healing needed to be broader. I was good on the practical end of walking out medicine, but Jesus wanted to partner with me in my everyday practice. Jesus wants in. He doesn't want to control us like a robot. We don't live like a mindless marshmallow or a sacrificial doormat. Jesus literally wants to walk through our day with us, advising us, whispering wisdom in our ears, reminding us of something we may have missed.

It's a partnership, but we need to know that our working relationship must be flexible. While we study, prepare, research, and care for the sick, he provides the wisdom, insight, and power, and carries the weight of the burden. Every day I encounter patients with complex needs, and it requires a lot of work to get them on proper medication, provide education, answer their questions, send referrals, and order the labs and diagnostic imaging. Jesus trusts me to uphold my end of the partnership. He doesn't always have something to say over my patient, but I feel his pleasure and his love for the care I am giving. He sits back and lets me do my thing. There are other times when he starts to speak and I need to let him take over the clinical encounter. There have been occasions when he waits until the patient has established care and then he jumps into the visit to provide the final step of healing.

I also have spiritual gifts that I can utilize in my profession, a truth I fought against for years in my old theology. Thankfully, spiritual gifts are available to each of us as Christian frontline workers who receive the sick. But how many of these gifts are dammed up behind a determination to adhere to medical science alone? How many sick patients miss out on a gift from the Holy Spirit because we've stubbornly rebuilt our theological barriers? That used to be me, and I'm so thankful the Holy Spirit helped me break down the dam of resistance so his river of healing could flow through me with his gifts. Superpowers such as the gift of prophecy or healing are powerful in the healthcare profession, and this was demonstrated during a recent clinical encounter with a patient.

My patient came to see me because of a lump. I could feel the firmness of it—hard and nonmobile beneath my fingers. I felt a little sick to my stomach. The ultrasound came back recommending a biopsy, which resulted in a diagnosis of cancer. I quickly notified the surgeon. A few days before surgery, my patient came to see me. I gathered the staff to join me and the patient in prayer for healing. We prayed for the surgeon and we prayed for a quick recovery after surgery.

Standing behind my patient while we prayed, I immediately received a picture in my mind of a scene from the movie *The Lord of the Rings*. I could see Gandolf slam his staff into the ground and declare the iconic line: "You shall not pass." I felt God say to me, "Rhonda, stand with the lymph nodes and say to the cancer, 'You shall not pass!'" The gift of prophecy can look weird to others, so I said it quietly to myself while the staff prayed out loud for my patient.

The surgeon removed the cancerous tumor along with several lymph nodes. A couple of weeks later, the patient called me with concern. It turned out that 75 percent of the removed nodes were malignant. The radiologist said it didn't look good. At that moment, I felt I should tell the patient about seeing the image of Gandolf and the words "You shall not pass!" during our pre-surgery prayer. I wasn't sure about this person's personal theology, whether something like this would be welcome or not. But they thanked me and told me that they were encouraged by these words. The patient had already felt like they just needed to hold on to faith.

I didn't hear from my patient for another couple months and then the phone call came. "Rhonda, I went for my final imaging. They told me the cancer did not pass through the lymph nodes! I don't even need chemotherapy."

I wish I could say I hung up the phone with confidence, saying to myself, "Yep! I already knew that!" but instead I laid my head on my desk and wept. I wept over my constant fight with believing the prophetic pictures that Jesus gives me, I wept because of the lack of confidence I have in walking this out in a greater way, I wept with thankfulness that Jesus would use me in this role, and I wept with thanksgiving that he took care of my patient. This situation is a good example of how we draw from medical science and the supernatural gifts that we carry.

FORETELLING AND FORTHTELLING

Prophetic ministry is both foretelling and forthtelling. This means that a prophetic word that comes from the Holy Spirit can foretell future events and provide insight or guidance about what is to come. But prophetic words can also be forthtelling words. This means the Holy Spirit speaks out or declares truths, insights, or even actionable outcomes. Prophetic words are powerful and can bring forth life.

In Ezekiel 37, God took Ezekiel before a valley of dry bones and asked the prophet if these bones could live. Ezekiel's answer was one of uncertainty. He could not foretell, so he replied, "Only you know that, God!" Later, God directed Ezekiel into examples of forthtelling. Ezekiel then spoke what he heard God tell him to say. It was not his own wishful thinking or something he hoped for or even tried to believe in. Ezekiel prophesied as God commanded him. His simple act of obedience in speaking what he was commanded to speak brought forth life and even courage to the house of Israel.

Jesus sometimes gives me prophetic words that are forthtelling, and these words come directly from the Holy Spirit who flows like a river from my belly. When these words come from the presence of God and we speak them aloud, they bring forth life. Prophetic words can also be effective in preventing harmful plans determined against vulnerable people. I have had occasions in my life when I have felt the Holy Spirit's disapproval and sense of injustice boiling within me. In these times, the pressure to release prophetic words comes from deep within my belly as a forceful flow of words comes forth out of my mouth.

During one of these occurrences, prophetic words changed the weather and canceled a large-scale event where young women were being exploited. On two other occasions, two separate buildings used for similar human exploitation were rendered useless by fire. No humans were harmed during these occasions, but evil purposes and designs were. Prophetic words that spring up out of our bellies are powerful, and it's important to recognize when God wants to collaborate with us to break through the gates of hell and advance the kingdom of God.

When I am seeing patients in my clinic and pause to listen, I don't always hear prophetic words over my patient. Sometimes it's wisdom, sometimes it's medicine, and sometimes people just need to feel seen and heard. My responsibility in this role is to listen to my patients and to listen to Jesus. There are days when it is so busy with volume and requests that I feel discouraged that maybe I missed something or didn't pray for someone or missed what Jesus was saying over another person. Despite my weakness and lack of confidence, I've heard him say, "Rhonda, it is spiritual and godly to do good medicine with integrity. This is just as important as prophetic words. You're doing a good job!"

One thing is certain: if we think we have a system or methodology to prophetic or healing ministry in healthcare, then we likely have stopped listening and have fallen back on a method. When Jesus healed, it was always different. He didn't have a methodology. He listened to his Father. He didn't do anything his Father didn't tell him to do. On one occasion his Father told him to rub mud on a guy's eyes (John 9:1–12) and the next time the Father told him to put his fingers in a man's ears (Mark 7:33–35). Other times Jesus interceded through prayer. It was always different, and this will be the way it is for us as well.

Routine medical protocol works because it provides familiarity, and we can do things automatically with or without God. In healthcare we run scenarios like cardiac codes repeatedly. The purpose of doing a CPR course every year is to provide an automatic standard that kicks in with repeated practice. Everyone does the same thing, and it reduces error and saves lives. It becomes automatic and systematic. We are able to take action without thinking or even having to listen. Doing things the same way places us in control during unstable situations.

While this pattern of automated routine may be necessary in medicine, it is not optimal in ministry. Our superpowers that we carry must be at the disposal of the Holy Spirit. This is how prophetic and healing ministry works. The flow of the Holy Spirit cannot be confined to a repetitive algorithm such as running a cardiac resuscitation code or the order of service in a local church. This flow can make us slightly nervous and anxious because we are releasing our own personal control over our environment, but releasing control is the only way the Holy Spirit can flow his river of healing from within us to a broken world.

Jesus must be at the center, and all we need to do is listen and do what he says.

CHAPTER 9
THE ART OF LISTENING

Listen to your patient: he is telling you the diagnosis.
SIR WILLIAM OSLER

I am a listener of stories. I think it is partly my personality, but I also feel that much of my ability to listen was developed by spending summers with my grandparents and taking part in family gatherings. Storytelling requires rapt attention from the listener, which was modeled to me as a child. Whenever someone told a story at family gatherings, the rest would listen and memories were made. I am a gifted listener. If someone tells me a story about their life, I easily remember it. It hangs on a nail in my brain.

When I meet a patient for the first time, I ask them to tell me their story. I always give new patient appointments longer amounts of time. This usually shocks people. They hold a list of their problems, expecting a quick visit—what one normally does when they go to a medical appointment. Unless there is an issue that requires urgency, I rarely deal with all the patient's problems on the first visit. In cases where immediate treatment is needed, I always rebook them later to hear their story and get greater details about who they are. I have found that a good story helps me to remember critical details about the patient. Usually, at the end of the visit, I have an entire history that stays in my brain. If I see an unfamiliar patient's name on my daily schedule, I quickly look in their chart and read the first few lines of their visit when they established care, and immediately I remember who they are and the details of their life.

The skill of listening is incredibly important. For some of us it comes easily; for others it requires work. Listening endears us to our patients, but it can also lead to other problems if we are not careful.

LEARNING HOW TO LISTEN

Not everyone is a good listener, but that doesn't mean we can't learn to be. Years ago I attended a conference in Toronto focused on community development. In addition to multiple main speakers, other professionals participated in an afternoon marketplace to showcase whatever community-building practice or gift they did personally or professionally. It was there I met a man called "The Roving Listener." He taught that listening was the key to community development.

In his demonstration, he shared how he teaches the art of conversation and listening. He trained an entire group of young people at a local church to go out into the community with a script to gather information for community building. The trainees went door to door, asking a series of questions to collect information about the people in the community. The neighbors loved sharing information with the young people. The young people then wrote the collected information on large sticky notes and stuck the notes on the basement walls of the church. They used the information they'd gathered to organize people into groups with common giftings and passions. Finally, they introduced members of the community to others within their groups of similar interests.

I listened to one woman explain that she had lived across the street from the same woman for sixteen years and knew nothing about her until she was told they both had a similar skill. They teamed up and became an integral part of a community group that brought hope to their neighborhood. Listening is powerful.

I enjoy listening so much that I can easily lose track of time. Unfortunately, this can lead to problems of efficiency in my primary care practice. My colleague's name is Nico. She is a friend but also works alongside me as a medical assistant. God knew I needed her; she keeps me organized and on time. If I get behind, Nico will knock on the door, interrupting the encounter to let me know my next patient is ready and waiting. This gives me a chance to end encounters politely so my patients feel heard but still understand others are waiting. Nico is gifted with organizational skills, and I need her to keep me on task.

Years ago, listening almost cost me my career in nursing. During the last phase of my diploma RN nursing program in 1986, I decided to complete it by training in a rural community so I would have a different experience in nursing. The hospital was in central Alberta, Canada, near a large Bible college. Many of the patients were elderly and frail former missionaries or Bible college teachers. Their inspiring stories revealed incredible faith-filled adventures and miracles. These patients deserved honor and respect. They were easy to love.

I found myself sitting at my patients' bedsides in rapt attention, listening to stories. Our story times encouraged both the storytellers and me, the listening nurse. Unfortunately, I started to notice I was irritating a few of the other nurses. They didn't appreciate the lengthy, feel-good conversations as much as the patients and I did. Even though I had finished my assigned duties, I was not sitting with the nurses on breaks but chose to sit with patients to listen to their stories. This seemed to increase their frustration because to them it seemed like I wasn't "pulling my weight" within the team.

I recognized the conflict and frustration of the other personnel, but instead of trying to make things better, I did what most anxious people do: I avoided them. I withdrew during breaks to sit by myself alone. On one nightshift during a break, I sat in the dark, alone in an empty conference room, when one of the nurses came storming in. "Where have you been?" she demanded. "We are out here working as a team and you're off by yourself."

I tried to explain that I was feeling some anxiety and felt intimidated, which at the time was probably the worst thing I could have said. She reported me to the nurse manager, and I was summoned to her office the next day.

The angry nurse manager, her red hair piled on her head in a loose bun, scowled at me across her desk. "How dare you tell one of my nurses that she intimidates you! Who do you think you are, coming into this hospital as a student, telling my staff that you have problems with them? They have told me you are not a team player. You don't help. You sit around and talk to people when everyone else is working hard."

Then she said destructive words to me that almost derailed me from who I am today: "You will never make it as a nurse. You are not cut out to be one."

I went home that day, only two months away from finishing my nursing program, determined to quit. I visited an elderly mentor who lived nearby and told him I was quitting nursing school. He encouraged me to humble myself, go back the next day, apologize and request feedback on how I could improve, and finish the course. I didn't know the possibility of my finishing was on the line.

Before I could apologize to the nurse manager, the college instructors called me in to talk. The nurse manager had already given me an unsatisfactory on my evaluation. This mark resulted in an instant failure on my course. Even though this was the first time I'd received any bad marks on any of my evaluations, I would not be able to graduate from the program without the manager changing the "unsatisfactory" to a "pass" on the last evaluation. Unstoppable tears and a sense of failure overwhelmed me.

However, I kept thinking about my mentor's counsel, and I determined to go back to the hospital the next day and prove myself. I apologized, with four weeks to go. I was going to do everything I could to change their minds and jumped in full force. I stuck to the other nurses like glue and did everything I could to prove I had learned my lesson.

On the last day, my manager called me back into her office. She said she had seen great improvement, then handed me a Hallmark greeting card with a snake on the front, its neck all tied up in knots. I opened the card to read "Relax . . . you made it." She laughed at the card and told me I had passed. I stared at the card in my hands, not knowing what to think as relief filled my body.

When I think back to this time in my life, I realize this difficult lesson taught me a few things:

1. Teamwork is important.
2. Physical demands of a job can become more important than listening.
3. Taking time to sit with patients and listen can appear to others like you are not working.
4. Listening to patients endears you to them but can breed jealousy and frustration in others.
5. Listening can be costly and slow down efficiency.

The ability to listen is incredibly important for healthcare providers, but it can also cost in efficiency, organization, cost effectiveness, and team dynamics. Listening can also be weighty and emotional when our patients share stories of trauma. Despite its cost, however, listening to our patients is critically important in our medical profession. Listening is one of the best ways to actively love people.

The potential conflict with listening is reflected in Scripture through the story of Mary and her sister Martha (Luke 10:38–42). The two sisters were hosting an event with Jesus as the special guest. This dinner engagement must have been a huge ordeal to organize. Running an event requires an incredible amount of energy and logistic skills. It requires planning, seating arrangements, menu planning, food purchases, food preparation, social interaction with the guests, serving the food, and finally the clean-up once all the guests leave.

Jesus did not come alone. He was likely accompanied by all his disciples and possibly their spouses and other followers. We often assume Mary sat in an endearing position at the feet of Jesus in a sense of worship and teachability, but maybe the house was so full that there was nowhere else to sit close enough to hear Jesus speak. Mary was listening. She was completely unaware of the frustration brewing in her sister Martha. Martha could not listen. She could not hear Jesus because she was not close enough to hear him speak, and her mind was unable to receive any of his words since it was consumed with the details of the overwhelming amount of work loaded on her shoulders.

Anxiety usually wants to blame someone or something else. When we are drowning in a sea of responsibilities, our tendency is to pull someone else into our chaos for survival. Martha likely felt over-whelmed by the immense amount of work it took to run this event. She eyed her sister who was doing nothing but listening and deter-mined that all the present chaos in her life was a result of her sister. There was no mention of the event plan in the Bible. We don't know whether Martha knew how to delegate or establish personal bound-aries in planning this large dinner. What we do know is that she likely felt invisible and unappreciated. Rather than pull her sister aside and quietly ask for help, she created a scene in public and blamed her guest for not caring and not recognizing the weight of this production that she held in his honor.

The answer that Jesus gave Martha has been preached for over two thousand years to those of us who are "careful and troubled about many things" rather than the "one thing." Martha felt she deserved a medal of honor, but Jesus told her that Mary was the deserving recip-ient of something that would never be taken away, and she earned this by doing something that looked like nothing. She listened.

So yes, too much listening can cause conflict. Listeners often appear to others like they are shirking the more important duties. But that doesn't take away from the value and importance of listening when that is the right thing to do.

I started my first job as a young new graduate registered nurse in Moncton, New Brunswick, in 1987. Roughly twenty years later, I attended a community meeting in the same area where I had started my first job. One of my friends wanted to introduce me to an elderly woman. I was surprised when this woman said, "I already know Rhon-da." I couldn't remember meeting her in the past. She began by telling a story about her mother who was in the hospital twenty years earlier after suffering from a stroke. She continued, "I met you in that hospital, Rhonda. My mother struggled with speaking after that stroke. None of the other nurses would take the time to listen to her because it took so long for her to get her words out to try and tell them what she needed. But you would sit with her while she struggled to speak until you understood what she needed. I have never forgotten what you did for my mother."

I walked away from that conversation in tears. I was thankful that twenty years ago, as a young, eager graduate nurse, I had listened to someone in a vulnerable, helpless state. As I reflected on my rocky start into nursing, I thanked God that I successfully graduated as a nurse and that I have never stopped listening since.

LISTENING RELEASES THE FLOW

Jesus was a listener. He spent a great deal of time listening to his Father as the source for everything he did. Jesus only does what the Father tells him to do:

- "I do nothing on my own authority, but speak just as the Father taught me" (John 8:28).
- "I have not spoken on my own authority, but the Father who sent me has himself given me a commandment—what to say and what to speak" (John 12:49).
- "The words that I say to you I do not speak on my own authority, but the Father who dwells in me does his works" (John 14:10).

These verses highlight Jesus's relationship with his Father and reveal the way he listens to him. They also show the importance of listening. If Jesus himself did nothing other than what he first heard from his Father, how much more should we be listening to the direction of the Holy Spirit who lives within us?

Jesus talked frequently about ears. I've often thought about his comments when he said, "Hey! You have ears, so use them!" Listening takes effort. It is an undervalued resource that often feels like a waste of time and a lack of accomplishment. Like to Martha and my fellow nurses, listening to Jesus may look like we are not doing anything, but this is far from the truth.

Listening is essential to the powerful flow of the Holy Spirit through us. God wants to release healing to our patients through special gifts such as prophecy and healing. Yet, hearing God's voice requires time and it requires practice.

Throughout my life I'd seen glimpses of the special gifts given to me from the Holy Spirit, but I didn't necessarily understand how to operate them. I heard God speak to me, but I didn't seem to connect his voice to my gifts. I have heard people say, "If it's a gift from the Holy Spirit, then you shouldn't have to practice it!" The church seems to have grace for someone practicing the gift of teaching, but when someone makes an inaccurate slip in prophecy, the same rule does not seem to apply. I'm not talking about blatant false prophecy but rather an innocent misunderstanding that comes with learning how to use a new gift. Instead of extending grace, the church wants to throw stones. In my forty-plus years of ministry, I have heard some terrible teaching and preaching that improved with practice. I've also seen people operating in their gifts from the Holy Spirit do the same thing.

For this reason, it is necessary for churches to develop training and mentoring programs to help Christians understand the gifts of the Holy Spirit. Discovering our gifts and stirring them up by practice helps us to mature and wield our giftings well. We learn by listening and taking risks and practicing.

There are many helpful training programs and schools available today, most occurring outside of local churches. I have personally spent two years in a prophetic training program called Emerging Prophets. The teaching has been extremely helpful to me in learning to hear God and to partner with the Holy Spirit through the gift of prophecy. Prophecy is simply listening to what Jesus is saying to the person in front of me. Revelation 19:10 tells us "the testimony of Jesus is the spirit of prophecy" (NKJV). The apostle Paul encourages us to pursue prophecy. He further explains why he feels this gift is particularly valuable above all the others. Not everyone is called to the office of a prophet, but we can all pursue this gift and practice using it.

Prophetic training classes are meant to teach us to listen and to act on what we hear. We often practice this through short activities where we practice or stir up our gift. In one of our classes, my instructor wrote a random number on a whiteboard away from view. She held up a book and said, "I want you to ask the Holy Spirit the page number I've written down on this whiteboard. If you get the number right, you get the book for free."

Immediately the number 178 kept repeating itself in my mind. I didn't try to get the number and I didn't pray for the number; it just dropped onto the movie screen of my mind with color and sound. As the instructor walked around the room asking the other students their number, I wrote 178 down on my sheet of paper. She finally came to me, and I hesitantly stammered out the number flashing in my mind.

Her eyes widened. Then I saw her smile as she turned the whiteboard around, displaying the number 178. She handed me the book, but I was given more than a free book that day.

I asked the Holy Spirit why he gave me the number. I felt I'd been singled out in a room full of prophetic people. No one else had received the number, and I didn't even try. I heard him speak clearly, giving valuable insight: "I gave you the number for two reasons. First to show you that the words come from me. You didn't get it by trying. You need to learn the difference between trying to get a word and receiving a word. Second, you need to know that I decide who gets the word."

As prophets we can only prophesy in part (see 1 Corinthians 13:9). This means we often only get part of the prophetic word. When we receive such an incredibly accurate word, we can begin to believe we are somehow special and anointed. To be honest, I felt that way after getting the correct number on the whiteboard. I felt special—so loved and affirmed. Several weeks later, though, we did a similar exercise and I failed miserably. I had slipped back into trying rather than listening for his words to drop into my spirit. I also failed to remember the second part of the very thing he had been trying to teach me. If I do not hear anything from him, it's not because of me; it's his choice and I may not be the person he requires at the time. This is why prophetic training is so important; it takes time and practice to listen and act on what the Holy Spirit is saying.

RELEASING THE HEAVINESS OF LISTENING

In John 4:1–26, we read about a weary Jesus. His disciples recognized he was so weak that he couldn't walk any farther. They left him sitting by a well while they went looking for food. Since he didn't have a bucket to drop down the deep well, he couldn't even help himself to a drink. He was thirsty, hungry, and weary, sitting alone beside the well when a woman came from town to fill her waterpot. Jesus was so weak that he asked her if she would give him a drink of water. This request led to a lengthy conversation, including prophetic words from Jesus that identified some painful areas of brokenness in this woman's life. While he drank water from her waterpot, she drank in the words that he spoke.

His disciples arrived with food just as the woman was leaving. They were amazed by a couple of things: first, that Jesus spoke with this woman who was obviously inferior to them, and second, that Jesus didn't seem to be hungry anymore. They asked each other if someone had already brought him some food. Jesus told them very clearly that he had meat they didn't know about, and that the meat he consumed was words that came from his Father. Jesus told us here that the flow of his Father's words through ministry to the woman not only brought life to the woman, but these words also fed and sustained him. The same is true for us. The ministry of the Holy Spirit also ministers *to* us as the Spirit flows through us.

Just like Jesus ministered to crowds of eager followers and Martha took on the task of hosting hungry people at her house for dinner, we have said yes to the responsibility of inviting the sick into our practices. Our days can be heavy and chaotic. I often endure endless tasks, sometimes charting my findings late into the night. These demands are necessary in our profession, no matter how efficient we are. But if we become consumed by tasks, we will become frustrated, exhausted, and bitter. If we focus on just getting through masses of patients, we will be overwhelmed, become anxious, and blame others for the chaos, while feeling invisible and unappreciated.

Listening can endear us to our patients, but it can also prove heavy and burdensome. We can get a lot of information and help our patients through the art of listening, but listening alone cannot propel our patients into hope.

After we completed the Emerging Prophets training, a small group of us traveled to California to attend a conference that brought all the students together to celebrate their accomplishments. While at the conference, Jesus began to speak to me about my family practice. He brought up the difficult patients who had experienced horrible trauma. I'd sit and cry with these patients as they revealed their heartbreaking stories. These were serious tragedies, motion-picture drama that left the victims broken. As I listened, my patients felt loved and heard. I would do all I could to get them on the right medications, refer them to therapists, and simply listen, love them, and help them to feel visible and heard. My reputation for listening and caring seemed to attract similar patients with complex needs. I was taking Galatians 6:2–5, which says, "Bear one another's burdens, and so fulfill the law of Christ," to an inappropriate level. I was bearing others' burdens all right.

Jesus spoke to me softly in the morning before the conference started. He told me it was good that I was so caring and empathetic. At the same time, I was not moving my patients forward into hope. This was Jesus's job, but for some reason I thought it was mine. I sat with them commiserating in their tragic stories. I grieved with them, cried with them. But I couldn't take them any further. I know it's right to grieve and mourn with those who weep. Jesus is there to heal the brokenhearted, yet Jesus was not talking about that initial compassion. As I listened to Jesus speak to me, I realized he was talking about our partnership in managing these difficult cases.

I tried to explain this revelation to a few ladies I was staying with at the Airbnb for the conference. I shared that I thought it was my spiritual duty to bear the burdens of others, and as soon as the words came out of my mouth, a giant wave of grief rose inside me. My mouth opened to speak but, surprisingly to me, a loud continuous wail came forth from my soul and would not stop. I bent over in mournful, agonizing heaviness as the awful wail continued. I could only take a breath between the lengthy sounds of grief. Memories of my patients' tragic stories filled my mind as each wail of grief seemed to rise into the heavens. I was a human modem, starting with a piercing screech followed by a sequence of high-pitched beeps and warbling tones. I was connecting to the heavenlies through rhythmic high-pitched screams while uploading the files of grief to Jesus.

This went on for several minutes. Two women attending the prophetic conference stood beside me and held me up while I convulsed with sobs. They looked on knowingly, holding me while patting me on the back as though soothing a baby. "That's it, Rhonda. Let it go. Good job. Let it all out."

I walked away from that encounter changed. I realized I had taken on the grief of the world, believing it was the spiritual thing to do. This was godly, I had reasoned. In truth, only Jesus can carry these burdens. It wasn't intentional, but when I became a receptacle of sorrow, I was saying that perhaps I was a better expression of God's love than God himself.

There is a time to grieve with patients and to hear their pain, but once we establish relational equity with a patient, we must offer hope. And we can't offer hope without faith in a God who can help them. When we sympathize with hopelessness, we are saying no to faith. Eventually these sad cases will drown us in a sea of burnout. Mercy and compassion are good and beautiful fruits of the Spirit, but when we can't offer hope, we have stopped trusting Jesus—our collaborative partner.

Listening to Jesus does not mean we won't ever get physically tired in medical practice, but sitting at his feet and allowing him to carry the heaviness of our practices changes everything. Our perspective shifts when we listen to Jesus. When we make space for Jesus to speak to us, we hear how to minister to patients, work becomes ministry, and everything changes. When we listen to him, we receive energy, and the life-giving power of the Holy Spirit flows from us to the sick.

CHAPTER 10
THE MEDICAL PRIESTHOOD

I do not feel obliged to believe that the same God who has endowed us with senses, reason, and intellect has intended us to forgo their use.

GALILEO GALILEI

I have returned many times to the vision of the priestly laborers hoeing feverishly in their dry, stony patches. The soil was parched and desolate. Why were they working so hard in a place that clearly had no water? They wore the same garments—a one-piece robe made of some sort of handspun natural fiber. A rope-like belt was tied loosely around the waist and hung a little lower over the right hip from the weight of a worn leather pouch filled with herbs, potions, and medicinal supplements. These struggling laborers were healers in priestly robes. It was a scene straight out of a medieval period film, and this made sense to me. Historically, the roles of priests and healers were combined. Priests were the bridge between the divine and humanity. Healing resulted from their wholistic treatment.

I studied the laborers from the pathway that led to the great Parthenon-like building. They didn't seem to notice me standing there watching them sweat and struggle as they worked their rocky garden plots. My gaze lowered onto my own ensemble. Although being the only woman in this vision, I was dressed the same as these priestly healers. My medieval fanny pack held the same medicines as the others.

I suddenly became keenly aware of my calling into the medical priesthood. A sense of divine vocation filled me with a sense of belonging and purpose. I didn't run to join the other priests. I had worked their fields already. Growth and life would not come from the barren ground. I was looking for something different.

Somehow I knew the answer would be found within the walls of the massive, white building. When I walked onto the porch past the towering pillars and entered the darkened doors of this awesome place, I found the water source I was looking for when I saw Jesus sitting at the center.

In ancient history, healers often served dual roles as both priests and healing practitioners, intertwining spiritual and physical healing through medicinal potions and spiritual rituals. This can be seen all throughout Scripture and is also evident in various cultures throughout the world today. There is a distinction in the source of power, however. Moses stood on behalf of God while Pharaoh had his magicians, Elijah had to deal with the priests of Baal, King Saul sought spiritual assistance from the witch of Endor, and the apostle Peter had to contend with Simon the sorcerer.

Undoubtedly, there is an alternative spiritual power source that comes from our adversary, the devil. Jesus frequently spoke about Satan. The name *Satan* comes from the Hebrew word for adversary, accuser, or opponent. Jesus calls him the Evil One and the father of lies (Matthew 13:19; John 8:44). The Holy Spirit comes with truth, peace, and freedom, and when he comes into our lives, he transforms us, adopts us, renews our minds, and gives us special gifts.

This is described well when Philip traveled to the city of Samaria and demonstrated God's power for healing, deliverance, and miracles that brought great joy to the city (Acts 8). While the Holy Spirit was moving among the people, the Bible introduces another character named Simon. The people all recognized Simon as "the great power of God" as he deceived people through sorcery.

Simon's use of an alternative power source gave him great prestige and celebrity status in the city, but when he saw the demonstration of the power of God, he quickly believed and was even baptized. Simon continued with Philip, amazed and filled with wonder because of the miracles and signs Philip performed. This incredible, ecstatic rush of dopamine came to a sudden stop once the apostles arrived on the scene. Simon witnessed something incredible. He watched as the apostles placed their hands on those who had received the word of God and were suddenly filled with the same power that Phillip had!

Although Simon believed and was baptized, it does not appear he was one of the individuals the apostles placed their hands on. Perhaps he followed Phillip because of the miracles and not because he believed the word of God. Instead, Simon thought about the upgrade this would be for his personal ministry. He asked if he could purchase the Holy Spirit. Peter was livid and publicly rebuked Simon, telling him that his money can die with him because he actually thought he could purchase the Holy Spirit with money. Peter told the sorcerer that his heart was not right, that he needed to repent from wickedness and ask God for forgiveness. Peter then said, "For I perceive that thou art in the gall of bitterness and in the bond of iniquity" (Acts 8: 23 KJV).

I like the word *gall* in the Old English version of the Bible because it is a bitter taste that is known to all of us who have been unfortunate enough to vomit. Gall refers to bile, which comes from our gallbladder and is an extremely alkaline substance that has all the necessary chemicals to combine with acids to digest food. The extremely bitter gall burns our esophagus and throat on its way out. When Peter rebuked Simon, he called him out for bitterness associated with jealousy.

James also talked about bitter jealousy: "But if you have bitter jealousy and selfish ambition in your hearts, do not boast and be false to the truth. This is not the wisdom that comes down from above, but is earthly, unspiritual, demonic. For where jealousy and selfish ambition exist, there will be disorder and every vile practice" (3:14–16). When Peter mentioned the bond of iniquity, or sin, he told Simon that jealousy had enslaved him.

Although Simon's response indicates some level of fear and

concern, the question of whether he truly repented is left unanswered. There are some indications in early Christian writings such as Justin Martyr, Irenaeus, and Hippolytus. These writings mention Simon Magus, who is thought to be the original Simon from Acts 8.[1] Unfortunately, this Simon is not described as a member of the early church but as a significant figure in early heretical movements and false teachings.

The story of Simon teaches us several lessons about superficial faith, pride, and personal ambition. It also shows us there is an alternative power other than God's Holy Spirit that was utilized by traditional priests, sorcerers, magicians, etc. These traditional priests understood the connection between healing through a role in the community that utilized a combination of medicinal knowledge and spiritual practices, and this was best demonstrated by the Levitical priesthood.

These priests could diagnose diseases, enforce public health guidelines, provide dietary and nutritional education, and implement sanitation and cleanliness guidelines. This holistic approach was based on the belief that true health required harmony between the body and the soul, and that spiritual brokenness sometimes worked itself out in the body in a form of sickness resulting in healing that included both divine intervention and practical remedies.

Christianity played a significant role in the development of early hospitals, and the vocation of nursing came from the humble beginnings of Christianity. Jesus's teachings of love and compassion for the sick, such as the parable of the Good Samaritan (Matthew 25:31–46) inspired early Christians to create spaces for organized care. The Christian belief in the dignity of every human being made in the image of God (*Imago Dei*) became the basis of care for all individuals regardless of their social status. This was a revolutionary concept in the ancient world. Healthcare was often reserved for the wealthy or those of higher social status.

One of the earliest examples of a hospital can be traced back to Saint Basil the Great. In AD 370 he created a space for care of the poor and lepers, and it became a model for hospital design and operation.[2] During the Middle Ages, monasteries throughout Europe served as centers for healing, combining spiritual care with medical treatment.[3]

The vocation of nursing became closely associated with women in religious orders such as the Benedictines, Augustinians, and later the Sisters of Mercy and the Daughters of Charity,[4] but it was really Florence Nightingale who is considered the founder of modern nursing. Florence Nightingale was deeply motivated by her Christian faith and felt nursing was a sacred calling and vocation to serve humanity.[5]

Over time the world shifted, and spirituality was pushed out of the healing business for several reasons:

1. Advancements in medical science: As the understanding of science and human biology advanced, the practice of healing became more specialized and evidence based. The connection between the divine and physical healing was fractured.[6]
2. Secularization: Over centuries, especially during the Enlightenment period, a gradual separation of church and state occurred. Medicine became secular and scientific while spiritual care remained within the sphere of religion.[7]
3. Institutional development: Universities and seminaries created formal training for both doctors and clergy. Medical science emphasized scientific methods and clinical practices while religious training focused on theology, pastoral care, and spiritual guidance.[8]
4. Professionalism: The field of medicine became professionalized and regulated. Medical practitioners required formal education, licensing, and adherence to scientific standards. Clergy members focused on spiritual leadership, pastoral counseling, and religious rituals.[9]
5. Cultural shifts: Societal beliefs and values began to emphasize rationalism and science as the primary means to address health while spiritual and religious practices were seen as addressing moral and existential concerns.[10]

We are part of a medical priesthood; we are the receivers of the sick. According to secular belief, our role has been fractured. I believe the spiritual will compete with the physical unless we intentionally reunite them through the flow of the Holy Spirit. It is important to understand that our need for evidence, our medical knowledge, and our experience in treatment should not be identified as a lack of faith or an evil partnership with pharmaceutical companies or medical treatments. The medical priesthood embraces healing through faith in God's sovereign power to heal however he chooses.

AUTHORITY TO CONFIRM HEALING

Medical professionals need evidence. Is this a lack of faith? Should we be ashamed when we ask for evidence? I have sat in healing meetings with bated breath while numbers of people testify of healings. I am looking for evidence. I want to make sure! People can get hurt, people can make wrong decisions, and we can promote unbelief and skepticism in the world if these healings are not real. When the older man at the healing conference told me my medical background was messing me up, I walked away from that conversation feeling rejected and ashamed. I had been struggling to believe whether each testimony of healing was valid, and something inside me wanted to make sure people were healed; others labeled this a lack of faith.

I recently spoke with a young woman who was testifying of miraculous signs and wonders that included gems dropping from heaven. I asked her if she had taken these gems to be appraised. She looked affronted by my question and appeared irritated. She responded with an accusatory jab back at me: "I don't need to take these to be appraised. I believe they are from heaven already!" At first, I felt a little ashamed for asking her that question, but as I thought on it, I couldn't imagine God being nervous about being asked whether these gems were real or fake. Do we think that the gems will disintegrate if we challenge them, or are we afraid our faith will?

Within my professional career, I have personally witnessed miraculous healing. I was in the operating room when the surgeon opened an abdomen and could find no tumor. He ended up closing the abdomen while complaining that the messed-up CT scan caused a needless abdominal incision. I have spent a night in prayer for a woman with a brain tumor. She was going into surgery that week, and I reasoned with God like Abraham in intercessory prayer: "God, this woman has several small children, and they may grow up angry at you if she dies." Repeated imaging prior to surgery revealed the tumor was gone. These are miracles. They have the before-and-after proof of healing.

I like before-and-after proof, and I don't think God minds when we put him to the test. During a clinical exam, one of my patients disclosed that she had a certain condition that required the same medication for years. She had run out of this medication and felt the symptoms that had plagued her for years were returning, so she was seeing me to get a refill. I asked if I could pray for her. She looked at me in surprise and said, "Well, I'm not a believer in God, but I do believe in positive energy. Yes, you can pray if that makes you feel better."

I laid my hand on her and prayed for healing. Then I advised her to get her blood work completed before starting the medication so we could see her baseline. She told me her levels were always high; they hadn't been low in almost fifteen years. The next day when her labs returned, I reviewed them to find her labs were completely normal. Medication was unnecessary. I called the patient to let her know.

Surprised at the results, she admitted she did feel good and suspected her imagination had led her to believe her symptoms were returning. I knew I could not bring up that perhaps God had healed her. Even my own faith was grappling with logic that this was a coincidence. But I had her previous records and her recent labs to claim this genuine healing.

This inquisitive, detective, evidence-based quality that involves careful assessment and examination is part of our unique identity. We should not feel ashamed of our need to ensure healing has occurred. This should not be viewed as a lack of faith but should be viewed as the authority to validate miracles.

I recently watched a documentary on the healing waters of Lourdes and the medical association that evaluates cases of reported healings using rigorous scientific and medical standards. The criteria to meet the qualification of miraculous healing includes evidence that the healing was sudden, complete, and lasting, and that it cannot be attributed to medical treatment or natural processes. The number of cases compared to the volume of people passing through the water since 1858 is small. This means that as of 2025, despite over 7,000 healings reported, there have only been 70 officially recognized miracles that have met the criteria in the past 167 years.[11] Is testing miracles a lack of faith, or is this a responsibility for those of us in healthcare?

When I think back to my vision of the river and the priestly robe with the small leather pouch hanging from my waist, I remember how Jesus blessed me in my vocation as a nurse practitioner. There was no shame in that encounter, only an affirmation of my identity as a healthcare provider and minister to the sick. God designed us a certain way and placed an authority or anointing to be responsible to examine and clear those who are sick.

Jesus affirmed this God-given authority and responsibility for priests (see Luke 17:14; Matthew 8:4; Mark 1:40–44). He told the individuals he has healed to go show themselves to the priests. Jesus certainly could have validated the healings himself, but he recognized the authority of the priests and their role in examining the sick and clearing them back into the community. This license to examine was granted to the Levitical priesthood; the details are found in the book of Leviticus. Just as the priests had a unique role in examining the community for signs of disease, they also determined whether people were healed of their illnesses. We should not feel ashamed or ostracized in our medical practice or in our faith community when we feel the need to examine and verify individuals are healed.

Unfortunately, our role in the medical priesthood may be pushed outside the perimeter of the church. The nonprofit practice where I currently work is on a course to deliver healthcare in partnership with Jesus. I am thankful I have the freedom in my clinic to pray with patients and to depend on Jesus for his part in our collaborative practice. Yet even though I am walking out my identity as a priest who carries medicine in one hand and the divine in the other, I find myself stumbling and faltering within the church.

I am pushing forward in my medical priesthood to release the supernatural into my practice, but I don't always feel the church is welcoming me into the supernatural. At the same time, I have encountered resistance to medical input within prophetic healing circles. Much like the Levitical priests, I believe we have a role to play in the church, often amid conflict when it comes to our identity in bridging the gap between medical science and the divine.

Our ministry as healthcare professionals partnering with the Holy Spirit may not be welcome in places that believe healing looks a certain way, and our need to validate and confirm healing may appear to them as a lack of faith. While attending a special Bible conference I was asked to offer prayer and prophecy to an individual with a physical disability. I felt God was encouraging her as a person with a disability to minister to others who struggled in this area as well. I heard God say she had authority and anointing in this area of ministry, but she looked at me firmly and told me she had received prayer a day earlier and that she no longer was disabled.

While I listened to her testimony with respect, it was very apparent she was still physically disabled. It is times like this that the supernatural meets the medical priesthood. I did not see a genuine healing, and I am certain my diagnostic clinical skills would not be welcome in this environment.

We may feel hesitancy from the faith community, but we also do this to ourselves. I mentioned earlier that we hold medicine in one hand and the supernatural in the other. We may not speak up and offer medical advice during a healing service because of the expectation of those seeking healing. We pray for healing but keep good medical advice to ourselves, only offering godly wisdom in the confines of our clinical practices.

My husband and I are part of a prayer ministry within our local church. We stand at the front of the church wearing lanyards around our necks with plastic tags that identify us as the prayer team. As the church congregation is dismissed, people can come forward for prayer. I listen to Jesus while listening to the church members' requests. I offer prayer, prophetic words, or prayer for healing. Several times when I have been asked to pray for healing, I've held back my identity as a medical priest within the church because it would not fit their expectation of the miraculous. People want instant healing for conditions associated with obvious lifestyle choices.

Rick doesn't seem to have this problem. One man came forward to ask for prayer for his back pain. The Holy Spirit gave Rick a word of knowledge—that this man worked in office administration and sat at a desk for several hours a day. Rick confirmed this with the man and then said, "I can pray for your back, but you need to start going to the gym to strengthen your core. This will heal your back pain."

As I have said earlier, healing occurs in various ways. Our identity as healthcare professionals gives us authority and license to walk out our medical priesthood without shame, even when this identity does not necessarily meet the expectation of the church community. Our supernatural side might be welcomed but the medical knowledge and educational side may not be, or vice versa. Discovering and walking out our God-given identities is powerful. When we allow God's river of healing to flow through us, we are released from shame. Being a willing participant in the flow of the Holy Spirit and understanding our identity in him brings us into our rightful place within the kingdom of God.

When you think of identity theft, you think of a hacker or thief who steals your personal information and does activity with your identity contrary to your personal choices. Satanic identity theft leads to spiritual confusion and distance from God. He does this by twisting Scripture, reminding us of disappointments, using social pressure, and even using cultural influences. The Enemy comes to steal, kill, and destroy. A stolen identity keeps us from the very thing that will bring us fulfillment and significance.

I am good friends with a woman who helps individuals discover their unique God-given identity through a curriculum she developed titled *Destiny by Design*.[12] God uses her in unique ways to help individuals to discover, unlock, and walk out their calling. She once told me about a young man who was gifted in dance. He was extremely creative, physically attractive, and gifted at physical movement. He came from a Christian family who recognized his gifting in dance. At a young age he was launched into a high-level ballet company. Unfortunately, male ballet dancers do not necessarily fall within most religious or cultural perspectives of masculine identity.

The ballet company invited my friend to facilitate her *Destiny by Design* training to their dancers. When she described the biblical role of dancers in the Bible, a powerful release of identity unfolded. She explained to the ballet company that the dancers and worshippers who often preceded the presence of God were strong and powerful men. These talented individuals with natural, God-given expressions of beauty have an anointing in heavenly worship and spiritual warfare. Their authority to lead the presence of God by dance and worship advances the kingdom of God by breaking open the gates of hell.

One of her activities in the training utilizes mediums such as clay or art to express each person's unique design. The young man created a male figure from the clay, repeating over and over, "I am a strong, powerful man." My friend told me later that this young man became one of the greatest ballet dancers within his profession. Knowing who you are creates a strong firewall against spiritual identity theft.

Whether you are a medical professional or a ballet dancer, your unique identity can be stolen. Satan is skilled in taking Scripture and directing it toward our identity. Our identity was also stolen from us when our priesthood was fractured. For those of us working in healthcare, a stolen identity places us at a distance from Jesus. Working as a healthcare provider without the flow of the Holy Spirit from within us places us in the rocky soil beside haggard priests, sweating under the hot sun in fruitless garden patches. We're not even in the building where Jesus sits in the center of the room.

If you are one of those tired priests, Jesus waits for you with cool, thirst-quenching water that will bring life to you and to those around you. We become powerful when we know who we are and take our rightful place of authority as a medical priesthood within the kingdom of God.

CHAPTER 11

AUTHORITY TO DO NO HARM

Do no harm, but never be afraid to speak your mind.
Harmful silence is the worst crime of all.
ELEANOR ROOSEVELT

Individuals with a strong sense of justice, well-being, and protection, and those who respect human dignity, are often called into healthcare. Money and job security may be a motivator for some, but this is usually not sustainable in the long run. Medicine is based upon the principle of "do no harm." This principle is foundational for those of us called into healthcare and is one of the four main principles of medical ethics. "Do no harm" is often referred to as non-maleficence and dictates that healthcare professionals avoid causing harm to patients.

When I develop a plan of care for my patients, one of the first thoughts on my mind is whether my treatment plan will be harmful to my patient. Being a healthcare provider is often very pastoral—with a desire to take care of people, making sure they are healthy and out of harm's way. For me, pastoral care is probably the focus of my profession. Prevention of harm, reduction of harm, and immediate safety from harm is an authority and anointing that falls upon us as

Christians who are called into healthcare. Looking back to the great room full of scrolls, books, and research that lined the walls of the room with Jesus at the center, I am deeply thankful for the advancements that have occurred because of individuals called into healthcare. I see global improvements as a result. Sadly, though, this perspective is not always shared by those we serve. Some seem to think their knowledge surpasses the accumulation of modern science.

Our nonprofit clinic provides both primary care family practice and urgent care services. Our urgent care sees hundreds of patients per year, some from the local community but many from various other countries who are visiting Hawaii on vacation. I work with excellent colleagues who give outstanding care, but there are occasions when the people we serve arrive with preconceived notions and expectations.

On one occasion, my colleague described a patient who demanded antibiotics for a diagnosis of a viral illness. When the provider told the patient they would not prescribe antibiotics, the patient became enraged and made accusations of incompetence and negligence. My colleague stood firm, but the onslaught of disrespect and unkindness left my colleague deeply hurt.

The overuse of antibiotics is a significant public health concern and has contributed to the development of antibiotic resistance, resistant superbugs, increased healthcare costs, and a global threat of resistant diseases. As healthcare providers we have taken on the authority to do no harm to our patients. This may mean withholding treatment that we believe would harm our patients.

I also have situations where I prescribe necessary treatment but the patient does not comply. Sometimes it's because of affordability, or inconvenience to go pick up a prescription, but for the most part it is usually because the patient decides the treatment will harm them. I am a big believer in the patient's right to refuse treatment. I always discuss the plan of care with my patient and advise them of the reasons behind this plan. Ultimately the follow-through belongs to the patient. I have learned over time that I cannot work harder than the patient. Regardless, this strong desire to pastor our patient from harm is the result of an anointing and authority that we as healthcare professionals carry on our shoulders, both personally and professionally.

Healing meetings are tricky for healthcare professionals. Many models or strategies in healing ministry have been successful, but if healing prayer becomes a strategy rather than listening to what Jesus is saying, this type of ministry becomes dependent on a method rather than the Spirit. This can lead to harmful experiences for others, and if healing does not come, it can destroy faith, cause disappointment, and lead to high levels of skepticism and unbelief.

I have personally been in meetings where several people testified that healing has occurred. I am not saying it hasn't occurred, but I feel it is important to test healing and validate it prior to public testimony. I have been in healing meetings where I have asked for prayer for a specific health issue myself. After prayer, the person praying for me asked me to test my injury to see if I was healed. I did and said no and she prayed again. After this happened three times, I was starting to feel inner pressure to say my injury had improved. There is something unhealthy if the recipient or the healer feels pressure or shame if healing does not come at that moment. We understand healing comes from the Holy Spirit, in his time and in his way. We can only open ourselves to his flow.

HARM VERSUS HEALING

Many of us have stories of encountering harm from medical interventions; we also have stories of harmful spiritual interventions in churches. One of my good friends, Gord, has been leading a prophetic ministry for years. One time we were discussing harm that has occurred through prophetic and healing ministries, and I explained the need for prophetic training and how I felt this could reduce harm. Gord agreed and added, "When the Holy Spirit shows up, you can't always control human crazy. If you try to control everything that appears crazy, you risk controlling the Holy Spirit."

My thoughts on harm reduction may have seemed logical to me, but I knew what Gord said was true. I have been in meetings where the room is thick with God's presence; genuine emotional and physical healing are happening; and revelation, direction, and acceleration of spiritual gifts are occurring over multiple people in various ways all at once. The air can feel electric, the presence of the Lord can make you feel drunk, and you can become charged with an ecstatic sense of joyous invincibility. We can become like Roy O'Bannon, played by Owen Wilson in the movie *Shanghai Noon*, when he says, "I don't know karate, but I know Kar-azy and I can use it!" This kind of "crazy," as Gord put it, makes us uncomfortable. We prefer being in control, keeping things orderly. Being out of control appears to expand the risk for doing harm. Do we risk shutting down the work of the Holy Spirit because we are afraid of harm?

Rick and I host a small group in our home. The purpose of the group is to focus on ministering and training others in prophetic ministry. We decided early on that this group would be an open group; we would receive anyone who walked in the door. The Hawaiian word *ohana* is a beautiful word for family; however, its significance goes beyond the conventional definition of family. *Ohana* symbolizes unity, trust, support, and respect. *Ohana* implies connection and mutual support. *Ohana* is a place where I can belong but also take responsibility for others. I believe there is no other word available in the English language that describes the kingdom of God as well as *ohana*. The word *ohana* brings forth Disney-like images of harmonious tropical family get-togethers where I am visible and everyone knows my name. First-time visitors see the harmony, but commitment to *ohana* requires vulnerability, sacrifice, discomfort, and risk. It means accountability, coaching, responsibility, and safe, loving teamwork.

We never know who will be walking into prophetic *ohana*. New people wander in every week. They usually come for various reasons: they are curious, suspicious, hungry, or desperate and broken. On one occasion a woman who was visiting the island heard about our group and wandered in to participate. She had lived in Hawaii in the past and had served in a large missionary organization. Prophetic words that were accurate were spoken over her that night. Feeling safe and supported in our group, she shared her story of the sudden onset of chronic illness while in full-time ministry. She described the emotional damage she encountered in healing meetings and the theological arguments that suggested oppression or a lack of faith. When asked if she would like to receive prayer for healing, she hesitated. I looked across the room at her, head bowed, lines of indecision and fear frozen on her face. We all immediately backed up to give her space. Having the group push forward for healing prayer for her chronic illness when she did not ask for it could be harmful.

I could see that this young woman needed healing, but not from the chronic disease we had zeroed in on during prophetic ministry. Instead, we listened to her journey that described the depths of intimacy, comfort, and deepened spirituality that resulted from strength made perfect through weakness. The healing this woman needed right then was more associated with personal trauma from methodologies and theological arguments that she encountered in the Christian community during a vulnerable time in her life. Right now, she needed love, acceptance, and a sense of belonging in a group of people who recognized that her identity was not a chronic illness but rather one of courage and strength to walk through it.

Perhaps love, unity, follow-up testimonies, and individual debriefing opportunities following ministry opportunities are the best form of harm reduction. Spiritual maturity takes time, and we all are human beings with baggage, in constant need of inner healing and personal growth. Harm happens. We can disciple and teach, but maturity, discipleship, forgiveness, restoration, and reconciliation are all necessary components of being healthy.

One of my patients received a diagnosis of cancer. I sent him to an oncologist who recommended chemotherapy. This man and his wife had been in ministry for years, and he prayed about whether to accept the oncologist's recommendations. Once he had decided, he shared with me, "I've had so many friends who decided to refuse chemotherapy and noticed that most of them died. I prayed and felt peace to move forward with treatment." I supported his decision and responded to his needs while he went through his chemotherapy. Their Christian community surrounded them with prayer and financial support, and he went on to finish all his treatments and continues to move forward in ministry today.

I found out later that his decision to take chemotherapy was met with concern, warnings, and shame—mostly from the prophetic community. This is a problem and it causes harm.

If I am honest, there have been times at our small ohana group when I have sat in a corner with anxiety, wondering if the meeting would go off the rails as we pursued prophecy. The church at Corinth is a good example of one that went off the rails. The apostle Paul took time to write long letters to the Corinthians to address their problems, including divisions, immorality, lawsuits, a misunderstanding of Christian liberty, abusing the Lord's supper, misusing spiritual giftings, and heresy. Confronting these problems in the church head-on took courage that most of us don't have.

Our first response to messiness is avoidance; it's a coping mechanism for anxiety. No one wants to deal with a mess. This is true for us walking out our spiritual gifts in our healthcare professions. We are fearful we will harm people, so we don't do it at all.

I have a sign in my exam room from the Disney movie *Lilo and Stitch*. It says "*Ohana* means family. Family means nobody gets left behind or forgotten." The people who come to us in church or in our exam rooms come in by invitation. When we throw open the doors to *ohana*, we are inviting in people with cultural diversity and influences, varying moral climates, immaturity, social stratification, and human nature. This can turn into all sorts of crazy, and our immediate impulse may be to pull back and control the crazy by shutting down the operation of the Holy Spirit. Our medical priesthood authority for harm reduction is good, but when it becomes Holy Spirit reduction, it has crossed the line.

While those of us in healthcare stop the flow of the Spirit flowing through our gifts such as healing and prophecy because we don't want to harm anyone, churches try to stop the crazy by using the confusion in the Corinthian church as a basis for concern. They focus on the crazy, unhealthy, harmful stories associated with the operation of the gifts of the Holy Spirit. Churches create religious security guards, thinking they are ensuring biblical order, rather than raising up mature coaches and mentors to facilitate the edification of the body of Christ. Although the church at Corinth had its faults, it had one thing right: it was trying.

On the home page of a church in Honolulu, Hawaii, I read the words *Faith means trying*. I have failed many times, but faith keeps me trying. Have we as Christian nurses and doctors stopped trying to practice utilizing our gifts from the Holy Spirit? Trying doesn't mean we'll always get it right. It just means that we'll get it right more often.

Trying means we need to take risks. Think back to the vision of the haggard priests frantically digging in the dry, unfertile soil, laboring under the hot sun. They were trying, but it wasn't faith. Faith means dropping the garden tool and running into the building where Jesus sits at the center. Faith means believing to the point that we act on what we believe. If we do not try, we will never see the promise of living water springing from our belly; we won't see the river of life flow to the dry and dusty places around us. Holding back the flow of God's river of healing causes harm. Allowing the Holy Spirit to flow through us brings healing. All we have to do is try.

OPEN THE GATE

When I began writing this book, I wasn't sure of God's objective other than the vision he gave me of the river springing up and carrying me to the world's medical library where Jesus sat in the center. I realize now that he wants to break open a gate into healthcare that has been locked. Gates require keys, and throughout history there has been an ongoing game of key snatching. Just like my illustration of the beaver dam holding back the flow of the stream, locked gates hold back the flow of the Holy Spirit. Here on earth, injured or sick people can find treatment 24/7 at a local emergency room, but there are spiritual gates found in Psalm 24:7 that need to open so the King of Glory can come in. David prophesies to the gates to open and be lifted. He says, "Lift up your heads, O ye gates; and be ye lift, ye everlasting doors; and the King of glory shall come in" (KJV).

Why are the gates closed in the first place? Why is David telling them to open? Who has the keys? Jesus talks about stolen keys in Luke 11:52, and he was not happy about it. In this passage he targets lawyers who were known as experts in Jewish law. The key of knowledge symbolizes a key that provides access to spiritual truths and a deeper relationship with God. Jesus said that this group of lawyers created their own set of legalistic and often burdensome interpretations of law. Laws are necessary and I am sure their system had many good things based on the laws of Moses and the Levitical priesthood, just as our legal system has some redeeming merits.

The real issue is that this powerful group took authority over justice and altered or created laws to maintain control. Jesus rebuked these lawyers for doing two things: first, they snatched a key that would open the door to knowledge, and second, they didn't go in, and they kept everyone else out as well. They didn't even use this key for their own purposes; they purposely stole the key to maintain control over the entrance. Power belongs to those who hold the keys.

Eventually this man-made group of lawyers that Jesus rebuked took authority over knowledge, giving them power and control over ordinary people. The very Creator of Justice and the Author of Mercy was pushed out of their legal system, leading to all kinds of injustice, and they eventually crucified the Son of God.

The same can be true for the gate to healing and good health. The 24/7 gate that David is speaking about in Psalm 24:7 is locked, and the key has been stolen by any group that maintains power and authority over access to healing without Jesus at the center. It is time for us to open the 24/7 gate so the King of Glory can come into our healthcare practices.

CHAPTER 12
RECOGNIZING THE MIRACULOUS

*Miracles happen every day, change your perception of what a miracle is
and you'll see them all around you.*

JON BON JOVI

Every time the medical ship pulled into a remote village in Papua
New Guinea, we were met by crowds of people seeking medical
help. I saw healing occur with medicine, I saw blind eyes see through
cataract surgery, and I saw infectious diseases prevented by education
and immunizations. These strategies are no less miraculous than the
laying on of hands for healing.

As healthcare professionals, we need to always have a sense of the
miraculous. The discovery of a test that detects colon cancer so
cancerous polyps can be surgically removed is a miracle. The rapid
tests we use to test for malaria are miraculous. When the surgeon
could not find the tumor that had been clearly identified on the CT
scan was a miracle. The miracle of healing surrounds us. We can have
the same response of thankfulness for the miraculous, whether it
comes through medication or prayer. Failure to recognize that every
good gift comes down from above will lead to an imbalanced view of

healing and an inability to receive instruction from the Holy Spirit who sits at the center of the room.

MIRACLES OF PREVENTIVE MEDICINE

In 2007 I was working as a registered nurse in eastern Canada where Rick and I had settled with our three teenage daughters and two sons and our dog after driving the yellow school bus across the country. That year a new vaccine was introduced specifically for girls between the ages of nine and thirteen years of age, for the prevention of human papilloma virus (HPV) infection. HPV is a virus that can cause an infection on the cervix of a woman's uterus. Over time, constant inflammation from the virus changes the cells on the cervix to become precancerous and eventually cancerous.

Cancer is basically caused by repeated inflammatory hammering on the cells of our body for lengthy periods of time. We see this in skin cancer. Areas on our skin that are repeatedly inflamed by the sun eventually feel like they've had enough and start to look and behave in an abnormal manner. The same is true for esophageal cancer. The acid that is in our stomach is extremely toxic. The special cells on the lining of the stomach are able to handle stomach acid, but the cells that line the esophagus are not the same as the stomach cells; they cannot tolerate the daily burn of stomach acid that occurs with gastric reflux. Eventually these cells change their shape and behavior and develop into esophageal cancer. Inflammation from an HPV infection can lead to cervical cancer, anal cancer, oropharyngeal (mouth and throat) cancer, vaginal cancer, and penile cancer. HPV also causes genital warts, and although these are benign growths, they can be uncomfortable and require removal.

Since the advent of the HPV vaccine, cervical cancer rates have plummeted by 65 percent in Canada. In some countries, rates are much higher. There are also several published articles about the declining rates of genital warts associated with the introduction of the HPV vaccine.

When the HPV vaccine was introduced to Public Health in

Canada, it was met with resistance and suspicion, especially from Christian parents. Some parents believed that vaccinating their child against a sexually transmitted infection might implicitly encourage premarital sexual activity. Moral and religious practices that promote abstinence believed the vaccine was unnecessary, convinced their children would adhere to their principles. Others felt there was not enough evidence to support the safety of the vaccine and chose to trust in their child's natural immunity to fight off infections. Vaccine hesitancy led many parents to withhold this vaccine from their children.

A well-known infectious disease specialist worked at the same hospital where I served as an RN. Everyone knew the specialist was a Christian and attended a large charismatic church in the city. I knew him to be a godly influence in the hospital. He was well respected, incredibly intelligent, and caring. He was quite disturbed by the attitudes surrounding the vaccine and began to speak out about the resistance to what he saw as a miracle.

During a presentation to promote the vaccine, I heard him say, "If we discovered a cure for lung cancer or brain cancer, there would be dancing in the streets! Yet here we have a cure for cervical cancer, and I am faced with a barrage of resistance and unbelief."

What do we define as healing? What do we believe is a miracle? Perhaps we need to rethink our definition of divine healing.

I have a Christian friend who is a high-level scientist in Canada and works at a university as both a professor and a researcher in science. She is brilliant and has incredible integrity in her profession when it comes to unbiased research. Her contributions to medical research and bringing evidence-based medications and treatments to the world look different from what we would account as spiritual. Her achievements look different from a healing conference where people cast off wheelchairs and crutches, but I suggest it is no less a miracle. As I mentioned earlier, failure to recognize the miraculous in the wisdom that comes from above can lead to an imbalanced view of healing. Jesus must be at the center of healing, and he guides us into all truth. The flow of a healing river begins with him.

MIRACLES OF PRAYER AND LAYING ON OF HANDS

On one of our inland outreaches from the medical ship, an ambitious young woman expressed frustration with the long lines of people seeking medical care. She wanted to be involved with the hands-on medical work, except she wasn't a medical professional. Rick and I listened as she expressed a desire to deliver babies and perform medical procedures like sutures despite not having any training in healthcare. My husband wisely recognized a call on this girl's life toward medicine. Rather than discourage her passion, he encouraged her to gather a few young people and walk through the lines of people offering healing prayer.

Over the next week I noticed the lineups were not as lengthy. We seemed to finish our days without sending people away. Every morning before leaving the ship, we started our day of outreach with a time of worship, a small Bible lesson, and some testimonies, followed by our game plan for the day. The medical team shared the statistics of numbers served, vaccines distributed, and dental procedures performed. Then the young woman Rick had encouraged earlier in the week spoke up. She stated that after being prayed for, many of the people asked, "Why should I wait in line when I feel better now?" The young prayer team's numbers of healings were in the hundreds, which had contributed to the reduced numbers of people waiting to be seen.

On another occasion a mechanical issue delayed our ship from leaving port, so our medical team decided to visit a local hospital. We walked through the building and prayed for the sick. I encountered a young woman on a hospital bed, groaning while holding onto her stomach. Her sister sat beside her holding her hand as I walked up to pray for her. I did not feel very hopeful for this patient. Without any faith at all, I did what was expected of me. The suffering patient looked up into my face with a look of helplessness as I placed my hand on her stomach and prayed that God would take away the pain and heal her body.

I walked away from this poor woman feeling so defeated. I could only think about the hospital's lack of imaging equipment and medical supplies. If only I could see what was wrong with this woman, maybe something could have been done for her. As we left the hospital that day, I felt my effectiveness was somehow suboptimal than when I worked in the lineups doing medicine. I couldn't wait to get back to doing medical outreach where I felt more useful.

The next day I remained on the ship to help with some of the ship duties while another team walked back into town for further ministry. Later they returned with enthusiasm to share what they had experienced. Rick found me working in the kitchen and couldn't wait to tell me about the woman with the abdominal pain I had prayed for.

"As we walked into town, the younger sister of the woman you prayed for came running toward me. She said, 'I've been looking everywhere for that White woman who prayed for my sister. My sister had pain for three years. She has been in the hospital for a long time. When that woman put her hands on my sister's belly, the pain went away. I've been looking all over town for that woman so I could say thank you.'"

I listened with awe, which immediately moved to skepticism. But how could I argue with this testimony? I did not have any faith or hope when I laid hands on this woman. It seemed surreal.

The testimonies did not stop. Rick went on to tell me what had happened at the hospital. The doctors and nurses told him that after our team walked through to pray for the sick, they were able to discharge most of the patients the next day since many were healed. I had worked with some of these nurses and doctors doing outreaches on the medical ship. Many of them were highly trained medical professionals who had taken their training in other countries. If they assessed the patients were healed, I certainly believed them.

The hospital administrator told Rick there was one hospital wing we had missed for prayer. The doctors and nurses in that wing were upset that we hadn't visited their ward for prayer. They saw how our prayers had emptied the rest of the hospital while they were still overloaded, with no available beds.

MIRACLES OF DIVINE INTERVENTION, SPIRITUAL PROTECTION, AND MEDICINE

Stories of praying for the sick without medical interventions can somehow feel more profound and miraculous, but as I have mentioned, healing can occur in various ways that are no less miraculous than the laying on of hands. During this same outreach in Papua New Guinea, I witnessed an incredible example of a divine redirection and spiritual warfare that resulted in a medical intervention completely orchestrated by God.

This outreach was a tight two weeks; the ship would spend two days in a village, then pack up and sail to the next remote community for another two days of clinic. These itineraries were established by the Department of Health, and we needed to be organized and rigid to maintain the itinerary. The ship always left on time, and villages knew when we would be arriving. Plans were scheduled weeks in advance so community health workers could spread the word that the medical ship was coming.

Like the father with his four malaria-stricken children with enlarged spleens, some villagers traveled for days to meet the ship. I witnessed one sweet elderly couple who arrived after a three-day trek over the mountains. The husband led his blind wife by the hand. She walked gingerly behind him, holding onto his arm with one hand while grasping a large walking stick in the other.

The ophthalmologist was only able to do cataract surgery on one eye. But she could see! I still have the image of her storming down the beach ahead of her husband who was now the one carrying the walking stick. She rushed ahead of him, excited to make the three-day journey home to her village to see her family—literally—for the first time in several years.

The ship provided dentistry, cataract surgery, and basic acute medical care. Our organization worked closely with the country's Department of Health to establish an itinerary for the medical ship. A group of their own national doctors and nurses partnered with us on the ship and took the lead in the medical outreaches. One key Papua

New Guinean doctor who accompanied us on this outreach specialized in tropical medicine while another key doctor was an ophthalmologist highly skilled in eye surgery. I was so thankful for their guidance and expertise, especially in tropical medicine. Foreigners like me walked in their shadows as we ministered to their people.

Villagers often welcomed the ship with celebrations in full tribal regalia and beautiful displays of cultural splendor. The air would resound with music and drumbeats as dancers performed ceremonial traditions. We felt humbled by their honoring displays of thankfulness.

On the last week of our outreach, we entered a village that felt different. The people sat in silence, subdued. They appeared to be controlled by one man who was covered with colorful paint and tribal dress. I watched my Papua New Guinean medical colleagues walking carefully, giving this man space to take charge of the ceremony. The tropical medicine physician who took the lead in this outreach had been trained in Australia, and it was so reassuring to have him beside me. Not only did he mentor me in tropical medicine, but he explained the cultural nuances, which were extremely important during our team interactions with local villages.

While staring at the man with colorful markings, he whispered, "This man is the *Tambuan* of the village." It became apparent this man held a position of spiritual authority. The people seemed to seek his approval regarding the ceremonial welcome and the scheduled medical outreach. The welcoming ceremony was mostly a one-man show as the *Tambuan*, accompanied by five or six other men, performed various ceremonial dances to tribal drums.

There was no sense of joy in this welcome. The villagers sat on the ground soberly while the group of men whooped and danced to tribal rhythms. There was a moment of silence and quiet whispers as men regrouped for a dressing change and returned to center stage in the middle of the large crowd.

My colleague stood beside me, quietly describing each part of the ceremony, relaying the meanings of each dance and setting expecta-tions for what would come next. At one point, they began one of their holy ceremonial dances where the *Tambuan* wore a triangular shaped costume with a dome-like cover on his head. His muscular lower legs were the only part of his body that was visible. He resembled a colorful Christmas tree with bare legs under a patio umbrella. The drums began their loud rhythmic melody, and four men around the *Tambuan* began to spin him in circles. My colleague whispered, "This is a very special dance for men. Women must stay back at least twenty feet from this ceremonial dance."

Just then, our cook from the ship arrived at the ceremony. She'd been delayed on the ship doing food prep and was excited to catch the tail end of the ceremonial welcome. This woman was an incredible addition to our team, full of joy and laughter and naturally funny. People loved her gregarious nature. She always drew a crowd, and God used her in beautiful, uplifting ways. The ceremonial regalia occurring in front of her was too entertaining and she couldn't contain her excitement, so she moved closer to get a better view. I watched horrified as she ran into the middle of the ceremony with her camera for a photo op.

The four men in charge of the *Tambuan* furiously pushed the spinning Christmas tree away from this joyful female trying to get a photo. As Rick lurched forward to somehow ease the situation, he could hear the cook laughing. Unaware of her cultural blunder, she was thoroughly enjoying her chase for a photo while asking, "How does he see under that costume?"

I looked at the Papua New Guinean doctor beside me, and he stood soberly staring at this cultural taboo. "It is good she is a foreigner," he muttered, "because if she was PNG she would be put to death."

After the ceremony we returned to the ship to get ready for a full day of clinic the next morning. The evening meal was excellent, we were all in good spirits, and the cultural taboo was forgotten by most of us. I lay in bed that night wondering about the blunder, though. Would this affect our work the next day? Would the *Tambuan* retaliate and cause problems?

The next day we loaded up the Zodiac, a rugged inflatable boat designed for carrying people, medical supplies, and gear to transport everything safely from the ship to the shore and made our way to the village. No one met us except the *Tambuan*. He wanted a medical visit from the doctors, but all other villagers were gone. We set up our equipment and tables, thinking villagers would arrive later. Only one man on handmade crutches arrived for care, crippled in one of his legs. We happened to have an occupational therapist from the United States and a physical therapist from Papua New Guinea who were able to help this man by providing exercises and new crutches.

When the afternoon rolled around, our team decided to change the itinerary. Clearly the people were staying away, and we didn't want to waste another day when we could be utilized somewhere else. My husband and the Papua New Guinean team agreed. We all felt we should leave for the next village. We could be there by nightfall and start our medical clinic a day early. We pulled anchor and sailed, arriving at the next village a day early.

Almost immediately, the local nurse came running for help. A five-year-old girl had been stabbed in the eye with a knife. The accident occurred when she tried to take the knife from the hand of her eighteen-month-old brother. Our skilled Papua New Guinean ophthalmologist, with some divine intervention, performed surgery and saved her eye.

I continued to see one patient after another—and then I heard screaming and shouting. A man with a machete started running toward the registration table. The young missionary volunteers who manned the table watched horrified as the crowd waiting in line jumped on the man, knocking him to the ground and carrying him off before he reached them. At that moment we received a call from the ship. A huge swarm of bees had landed on the ship, wreaking havoc on the kitchen operations. Thankfully the captain was able to chase the bees away with a water hose.

The day was exhausting, and after finishing the first day of clinic, our volunteers were tired, hot, and sweaty. When we had arrived, the local leaders warned us to avoid swimming near the mouth of the river where our ship was anchored. Two weeks earlier a pregnant woman had been washing her laundry on the shore when a large crocodile grabbed her and dragged her into the water never to be seen again.

Despite the warnings, the water looked inviting, our team was exhausted, and the rules were thrown out the window. One by one the team ran into the cool, inviting water for a dip.

Later, after I finished my dinner on the ship, I stood by the sea door's large opening and scraped my chicken bones into the ocean. (The sea door is a large metal door on hinges that can be closed watertight while the ship is underway and is opened to be used for embarking and disembarking the ship while docked or at anchor.) The light from the sea door shone out upon the dark water and I could see dim lights on the distant shore.

A flash of light caught my eye roughly fifty yards from the sea door. At first, I thought it was a tin can floating in the water, but as I looked closer, I realized it was a set of eyes watching me scrape my plate. There were crocodiles in these waters.

I walked back to the team to make sure no one went for a late-night swim and also told them to be careful to scrape the food off their plates from a higher location than the sea door, then asked the crew to close the door for the night. I didn't know if these things could jump into the ship from the sea door, but I didn't want to find out.

A few moments later, village leaders pulled up aside our ship in a large yellow banana boat. They were searching for a dangerous local who was suspected to have boarded our ship. This man was known for taking advantage of women. As they searched each room of the ship, they found their man in the ship lounge wearing a lanyard, pretending he was one of the Papua New Guinean medical volunteers on the ship. I watched as the officials and their prisoner shot across the water into the darkness back to their village.

This day had been incredibly crazy. My head was spinning with all the near misses of drama that could have ended badly, and I went to bed early anticipating a big day in the morning. It seemed I had no sooner fallen asleep when Rick came barreling into our cabin and shook me alert. "Rhonda! Get up! You've got to see this!"

I followed him curiously onto the back deck. The scene before me was surreal. Was I still dreaming? A black, squawking circle of hundreds, if not thousands, of birds were circling the ship, a tornado of red-eyed black birds. I couldn't believe what I was seeing. Birds were everywhere. They were on the aft deck where our team met for meals and they were in the bathrooms, but most of them were flying in their bird tornado. The birds gradually dispersed as daylight started to emerge on the horizon.

I hadn't yet pieced together that all the incidents, the nervous energy in the crowds, the bees, and the birds were possibly related to supernatural forces at play. It wasn't until later that I suspected it may have been connected to the angry *Tambuan* from the previous village. I don't know. But what I do know is that God's protection covered us like a supernatural sphere. He kept a madman from attacking our young volunteers. He redirected an angry swarm of bees. He shielded a tired medical crew from man-eating crocodiles. He thwarted the efforts of a potential rapist. Supernatural protection covered our team from sinister forces.

Miracles happened. We moved a day early to the next village, where God wanted to restore a young girl's eye. The surgeon told us that the surgical procedure would not have been possible if we had delayed our arrival by one day. God moved heaven and earth for this young girl to have eye-saving surgery, and it occurred through a surgical procedure performed by a highly skilled Papua New Guinean ophthalmologist who just happened to be on our medical team.

All of heaven comes to earth when we partner with Jesus. And as healthcare professionals, we are in a good place for Jesus to do the miraculous. We may not see the entire story of the miraculous depths God has engineered to bring the patient before us, but our skill, our medical knowledge and insight, may be the miracle this person needs.

THE MIRACLE OF PARTNERSHIP

I once had a patient who was suicidal because of severe pain associated with a chronic condition. He had been off medications for a year and was now in dire need of emergency treatment. I made him promise me he would not commit suicide until he gave our team a chance to get hold of his pain and treat his conditions. I ordered labs, placed him back on several medications, and made a referral for diagnostic testing. I also managed to convince him to make some lifestyle changes and urgently got him in to see three specialists. I collaborated with the specialists daily, and prepared and cleared the patient for surgery in less than a week.

One week post-op, my patient's pain was significantly reduced but the surgeon was still concerned. The post-surgical site was not healing properly. The surgeon determined the issue would require further extensive surgery.

Jesus was often moved by compassion, and I felt compassion stir in my spirit. I had done all I could do medically for this patient. As this man sat in my examination room, likely facing another surgery, the Holy Spirit indicated to me that he wanted to jump into the visit with his power to heal. I asked my patient if I could pray over the area that required healing and he gladly agreed. I prayed exactly what I heard Jesus tell me to say. It involved speaking to a part of the body that was largely responsible for this man's issue. Nothing unusual happened, though, and the patient returned home. The next week my patient returned and reported that further surgery would not be required. Post-op healing was happening.

This example demonstrates the beauty of partnering with Jesus in our practices. Both Jesus and I partnered in this case. The work I did on this patient was necessary, important, and still miraculous. The medications, the alleviation of pain, the sense of love and concern from our team, and the surgical procedure are miracles and wisdom from above. The suicidal ideation was gone, the patient felt loved and heard, and the pain was controlled. The transformation was evident. My patient's face reflected a look of peace and hope for the future.

If I didn't know how to listen, if I didn't believe there could be more, if I didn't believe in prayer for healing, and if I felt I didn't have the authority or skill to pray over my patient, then I wouldn't have given Jesus an opportunity to release his river of healing. If I hadn't partnered with Jesus, the outcome for my patient might have been tragically different.

CHAPTER 13
THE CALL

Fortune favors the brave.

PUBLIUS TERENCE (AND MATT DAMON)

J esus wants to partner with healthcare professionals. The study, the research, and the educational preparation are a necessary foundation that Jesus wants to use. He says that this is all good. We see the fruit of medical science and the incredible advancements that have been brought into the world. All of this is good and as James affirms, "Every good and perfect gift is from above, and comes down from the Father of lights, with whom there is no variation or shadow of turning" (James 1:17 NKJV).

As we've explored, there is so much more for us than can be contained in a professional medical degree. We are positioned strategically in the kingdom to bring forth a river of healing to the world. We are a royal priesthood of healers and not just healthcare providers. We stand in the gap between the divine and the physical. We are not practicing without a license, but we do need to practice our spiritual gifts with just as much dedication as we did at our earthly universities.

If we start and stop with medical science (which is still good!), we will be like the foot care physicians employed by King Asa. King Asa started his reign enthusiastically with dedication and strong leadership. He made hard choices and even stood against family members to follow God. But when a prophet called him out on his self-reliance, King Asa became so angry that he shot the messenger. After this, King Asa developed an "exceedingly great" disease in his feet and instead of turning to God ran to his physicians (2 Chronicles 16:12).

There are amazing physicians who carry great wisdom and experience but do not carry the supernatural insight from the Holy Spirit. King Asa's physicians were likely the best in the kingdom and highly skilled in medicine, but their efforts were futile. If they had partnered with God, they would have recognized that the root cause of King Asa's disease was not a physical one. It was a spiritual problem based in pride and bitterness. In this case the remedy would not be found in medical science, and in Asa's health crisis these physicians proved worthless.

The health advice to Job also proved worthless. Job uttered the phrase "worthless physicians" while in a severe mental health crisis (Job 13:4). He compared his close friends to physicians of no value. Their mental health response team gave counsel that did not come from the Spirit of God.

Clearly, physicians are good and necessary. Even Jesus said that sick people need physicians: "Those who are well have no need of a physician, but the sick" (Luke 5:31 NIV). This verse goes deeper than the physical needs of people. Jesus's statement was a shout-out to the Pharisees who considered themselves righteous and without need of spiritual care. They were blind to their own spiritual sickness. While physicians may take care of the physically ill, it is the Great Physician who uncovers both physical and spiritual sicknesses and brings healing to both.

There have been many times when I have been a worthless physician. I have spent exhausting years hoeing dry ground without the river of life flowing from within me. I wanted more; I was faint and thirsty, sometimes wanting *more* springs from a place of burnout and devastation. It takes time to rise from the places of skepticism, disappointment, and burnout in healthcare.

This book ends with a call to those of us who are called to the medical priesthood but feel impoverished. Poverty leads to hopelessness, stress, and burnout. We see this in the Bible when the Midianites prevailed over the children of Israel. Israel was greatly impoverished, and they cried out to the Lord for more. All their work efforts to get ahead and be fruitful were futile. Even though God sent a prophet to explain to them why they were in this situation, it seems he still heard their pitiful cries for more. In turn God raised up an individual full of discouragement and skepticism.

Gideon was called out by an angel, although he didn't seem to recognize the messenger as an angelic being. He dismissed the angel's affirmations and argued common existential questions about human suffering and even scoffed at the idea of miracles: "And Gideon said unto him, oh my Lord, if the LORD be with us, then why is all of this befallen us? And where be all his miracles which our father told us of, saying, Did not the LORD bring us up from Egypt?" (Judges 6:13–14 KJV).

Gideon was tired of hearing the stories of miracles. He had only heard about them but had never experienced one for himself. Despite his disappointment, a spark of hope was ignited in Gideon, and he asked for a sign. He asked the angel to stay put so he could run home and prepare a present. This present was costly for an impoverished family.

When Gideon returned, the angel was still there. The angel accepted the present and told Gideon to lay it on the rock and pour out the broth. I wonder what Gideon thought about that. Despite doubts, he obeyed. Somewhere in the back of his mind there was a memory of a story from the past. It shined a small glimmer of hope that seemed to move him forward in an act of faith. Gideon followed what he knew was the right thing to do. Even though he had never experienced a miracle for himself, he tried. Faith means trying. It means pushing past impoverishment, hopelessness, stress, and burnout, hoping for more.

Finally, the angel of the Lord put forth his staff and touched the meat on the rock. A burst of fire came from the rock and burned up the sacrifice. Typically, when fire shows up in the Bible, it is usually because of fear. Moses saw a burning bush, and the disciples cowering in the upper room saw tongues of fire. The fire of the Lord is the love of God, and perfect love casts out fear. After the fire consumed the sacrifice, Gideon heard the voice of God for himself. He continued to have moments of self-doubt and insecurity, but he still moved forward in faith.

The story comes to a climax when God tells Gideon to put out a call that is answered by 32,000 volunteers. God allowed the fearful to opt out, and 22,000 people took advantage of this golden moment. And then there were 10,000. God still said the number was too high, told Gideon to take the remainder to the water, and said, "I will try them there." The final cut of 300 people was based on the way they drink water.

This story has always left me with questions. It has never seemed very fair to me. There are several suggestions for why God chose one group over the other. Most teaching suggests that Gideon's 300 were selected because their drinking stance showed a readiness for attack, but I am not so sure. It is interesting to me that God chose those who use their hand to lap like a dog. I wondered if there was a symbolic reason for choosing the hand lappers, but I think the choice had more to do with those who fell to their knees to drink. Feeble knees are associated with becoming fainthearted and weak (see Hebrews 12).

As I thought about the 9,700 soldiers who dropped to their knees and faceplanted to drink, I remembered my husband Rick's story about the thirstiest time in his life. Rick is well-known for being a one-man team. He takes on challenges with a positive outlook, has incredible physical endurance, and usually runs out the door into physically demanding projects, underestimating the amount of time and energy required to complete the job.

This time occurred during one tree planting season in northern Canada while we ran the silviculture program. Rick needed to take our boat eight to ten miles across the lake to uncover a cache of frozen trees. During the winter, boxes of trees were covered with snow and then sawdust to insulate the frozen stock until it was ready to be planted early the next summer. Although the summer temperatures rose during the day, the trees remained encased in snow and ice.

Rick stood helplessly in front of a mountain of trees the size of a large two-story home, holding a small shovel and kicking himself for not bringing extra help. He needed the cache boxes to thaw by the end of the week, so he started shoveling. He encouraged himself that it would get easier once he reached the boxes but soon realized the boxes were frozen together. They needed to be pried apart before he could fling each fifty-pound box away from the mountain of snow. Rick had underestimated the time it would take to complete the job, and found himself feeling a little desperate as he stood there under the hot sun, covered in a combination of sweat, snow, and sawdust.

Rick told me later that he had never felt such thirst in his entire life. He grew weaker and more faint with each passing hour. He shoveled with urgency and came to the last layer of boxes. Seriously dehydrated, Rick stumbled back to the small boat. He wondered if he was going to pass out, but he managed to walk into the water, drop to his knees, and faceplant into the cool northern lake. No hands were used to lap this water; this was a full-on, knee-bend faceplant. With his head below the surface, he sucked in mouthfuls of cool water until his thirst was quenched.

I believe the final cut for Gideon's army was more about alleviating the faint of heart than it was about the stance and posture of the 300 that remained. The story of Gideon is a story about a discouraged and skeptical man whom God called forward as a leader to bring victory to an oppressed and impoverished people group. Those who would join the battle and experience the miraculous were chosen by the way they drank water. It is also a story about leaving the fearful and fainthearted behind. God calls those who want more.

There is a call for those of us working in healthcare who want more. God told Gideon he would try the people "at the water." The same challenge is there for us today.

Jesus wants to partner with healthcare providers to bring the divine back into our practices. We are members of a royal priesthood of healers, and we are meant to bridge the physical with the spiritual world so that healing flows like a river into the dry places of healthcare.

God wants us to seize our authority in the medical priesthood within our practices and within the church. There is a river to be released that comes from within you. You can experience the miraculous for yourself. It's time to walk past the tired, worn-out, priestly laborers. It's time to enter the cool medical library of fame and walk past the impressive volumes of books to the One who sits at the center of the room. He waits with cool water that he will pour into your hands to drink. If you ask him to touch your hands so that you can heal the sick, he will do that just for you. You already know that you have that gift. It is just ragged and hidden beneath years of painful discouragement, skepticism, and hopelessness. It's time for the river to flow again. It's time to stir up your God-given gifts.

I recently attended a large conference of roughly 3,500 people. We gathered to worship and to hear major Christian leaders who walked in the flow of the gifts of the Spirit. I was feeling rather dry spiritually, so I took some time away from my busy family practice to attend. I needed to be there. The worship encouraged me, and the stories of miracles and healings inspired me and increased my faith.

Every morning, groups of people from similar geographical locations were assigned together and met for a small pep talk and prayer. Each community group had roughly twenty-five to thirty participants. Our group contained those of us from Hawaii along with people from the West Coast. I got to know the older couple beside me as they described their denominational background, which was very similar to mine. They confessed they were a little nervous about attending this conference, and I laughed and told them that I could relate. Our conversation came to an end as the group leader pulled us all together.

Suddenly the older man beside me collapsed. Most of our team thought he was having a spiritual experience, but I knew different. I got down on my knees beside him to assess his condition. He responded to me and told me he felt dizzy. I went through a string of questions with his wife about his health condition and medications.

He seemed to improve, so we propped him up to a sitting position and got him a glass of water. I kept talking to him while checking his pulse. He was growing more confused, and his pulse was getting weaker and slower by the minute. Then he stopped responding to my questions. His heart stopped. I watched his face turn gray as his head dropped to the side.

I shouted to the ministry leader to call 911. She looked at me in surprise and said, "Really?", but then grabbed her phone to call when she realized the seriousness of the situation. As I got ready to start CPR, the leader told everyone to pray.

When I laid my hand on his chest, I felt the familiar weight of the Spirit, like the draw on the water pump back on The Hill, when you sense the flow of water coming up from the depths of the well. I can only describe this as a sensation of urgency combined with indignation that comes from inside and must flow out with some sort of action. I heard myself say an anguished and pleading prayer: "God, no! Not here! Not now!" I repeated this urgent cry three times. At the time I didn't know why I said those words, but now I think I felt it would be a shame for a man to die in the middle of a conference filled with people who believed in the supernatural power of healing. It would get around the community. People would remember a body being carried out of a healing conference.

I didn't need to start CPR. Within moments I could feel the life-giving flow into the man's chest beneath my hand. I felt his heart begin to beat, and he became responsive to my questions. I watched the color return to his face as the ambulance arrived and the paramedics rushed into the building. After I gave them a short report, I walked away from the crowd to let the EMTs do their job.

I kept the information about his heart stopping to myself out of respect for privacy. This situation didn't need to be shared from the public platform. This couple was new to this type of environment and I didn't want to cause added fear around his heart condition. I was in a confusing muddle of thoughts, so I wandered off alone and sat by myself. Shaking from the ordeal, I started to cry and flood God with questions.

What just happened?

Why did you place me beside this man?

Why did those words come out of my mouth?

Why did I feel a l forceful flow of power come from within me?

How come this didn't happen at other times when I'd laid hands on godly people who still passed into eternity?

I cried tears of gratefulness mingled with a thirst for God to use me more. After a few moments alone, I composed myself and wandered back to see the older couple still sitting in the same place with the paramedics. The man's vitals were normal and everything seemed fine. He refused to go to the hospital, insisting he felt okay. Later that day, I noticed him and his wife strolling outside during the lunch break.

This miraculous heart-stopping-and-starting experience was a revelation for me. I had seen people healed in the past, but this was on a different level. As I thought about this situation, the Holy Spirit began to remind me of other times throughout my life when I had felt that same sense of urgency, that same indignation that had led to miraculous events.

He reminded me of the time when our medical ship was being blown into the rocks by strong winds. The captain was helpless; he had tried to navigate the ship off the dock, but the strong wind had managed to parallel park us between the dock and another ship lined with nervous-looking men only twenty-five to thirty feet in front of us. We were boxed in and moving sideways into the rocks. In an emergency attempt to turn the bow into the wind, the captain sent my husband out in the dinghy to act as a bow thruster. I watched as Rick opened the throttle of the outboard motor pushing the dinghy against the starboard side of the bow. I could hear the roar of the ship's engine as the captain threw the propeller from forward to reverse in a last-ditch effort to turn the bow to port and avoid hitting the ship in front of us. All I could see was Rick's dinghy moving backward and the men on the ship in front of us wildly waving their arms, shouting orders, and running toward the helm of their ship.

I ran downstairs into my cabin and fell on my knees. The familiar sense of urgency rose up inside of me. I cried out, "God, send your angels to push on the side of the ship!"

Instantly, I felt a powerful jerk followed by a forceful steady movement from the starboard side. The ship was literally doing the impossible by moving sideways into the wind. It moved sideways until the captain was able to turn the bow into the wind and past the ship in front of us.

As I reflected on these experiences with the Holy Spirit, I realized he wanted me to learn and understand some important lessons: first, that I need to always remember the sensation and feeling of the weight of his presence and the flow of living water from within me, and second, that I have the gift of miracles. I was a little awestruck at that and told him I didn't feel like I deserved such a glamorous gift. That glitter faded when he tenderly answered me, "Rhonda, you need to remember that having the gift of miracles means you will be placed in situations that require a miracle."

This book is about the rivers of living water that can flow from within us to a hurting world. As Christians working in the world of healthcare, we have an incredible opportunity before us. I spoke in earlier chapters about blockages and barriers such as disappointment, doctrines, theology, and science that can create barriers to the flow of the river of life. Once we pull out those dams that block the river, we can start to feel and experience the flow that comes from within us through the special gifts he has given us.

We all have the wells of living water within us, but for many of us, a lot of energy is spent pumping air. Priming the pump is an act of faith that water will come. We may need to take a few trips to the water barrel, but this is where it must start. The Holy Spirit is the living water. It is his power that flows out of us. He wants to co-labor with us and through us. Over time, as we grow in experience and confidence, we can hear him more clearly, sense his presence more keenly, and partner with him through the special gifts he has given us. We can see the miraculous. The journey starts with one small step forward.

Jesus said, "Let anyone who is thirsty come to me and drink" (John 7:38 NIV). And, "Whoever believes in me, as the Scripture has said, rivers of living water will flow from within them" (v. 39 NIV). By this he meant the Spirit, whom those who believed in him were later to receive. Up to that time the Spirit had not been given since Jesus had not yet been glorified.

Jesus sits at the center of every piece of wisdom that has come down from the Father of lights and says, "All of this is good, but keep me at the center."

Through the years . . .

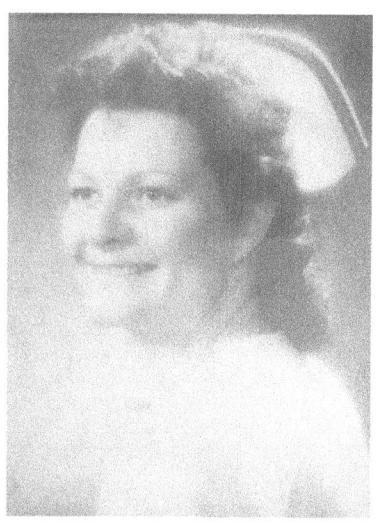

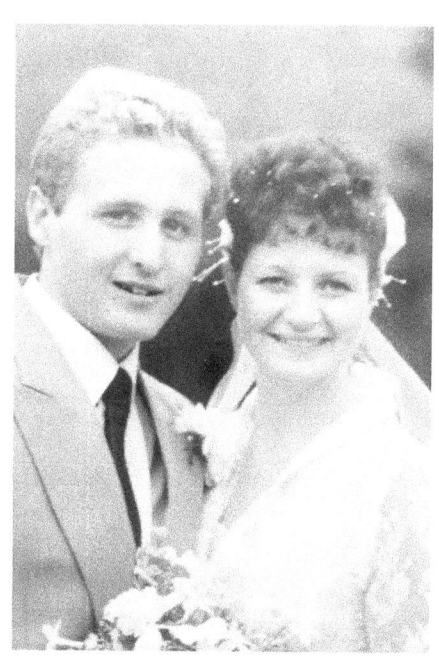

Nursing school graduation, 1986   Rick & Rhonda's wedding, 1987

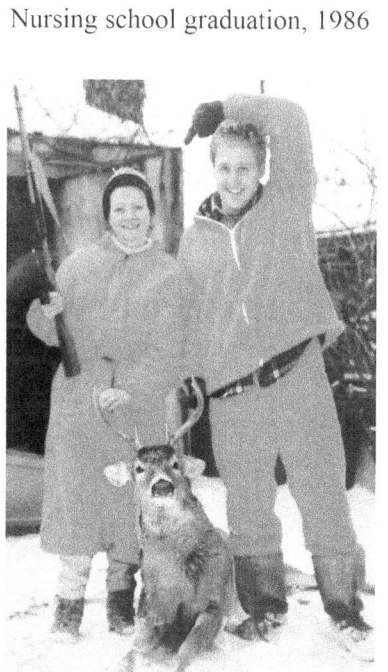

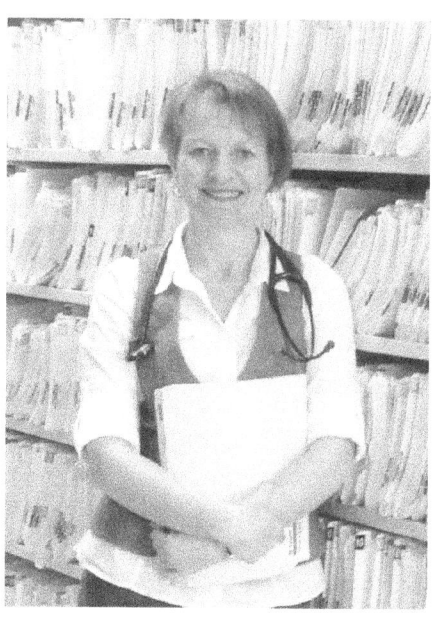

Deer hunting in the early years   First nurse practitioner position, 2013

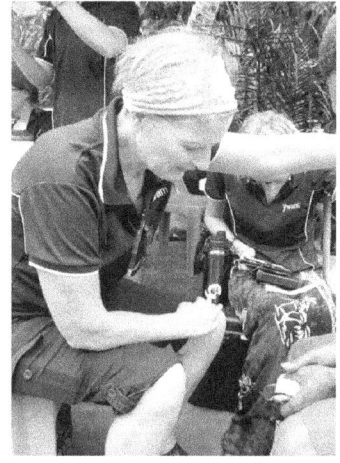
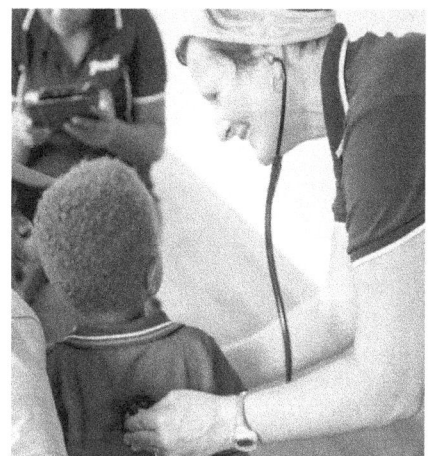

International Medical Missions

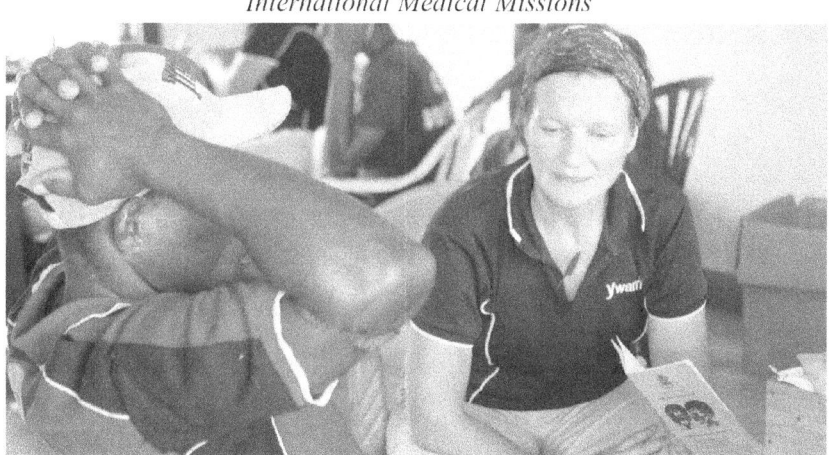

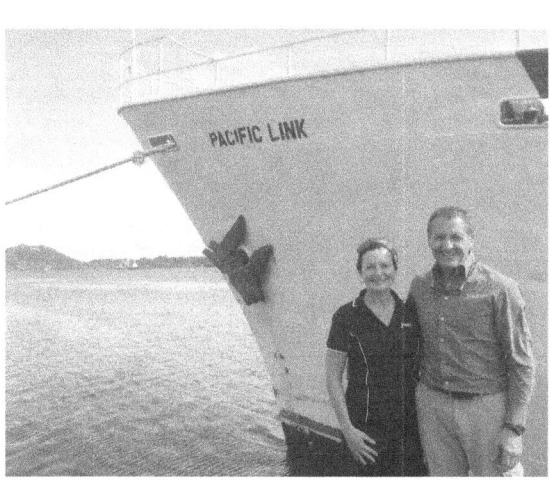
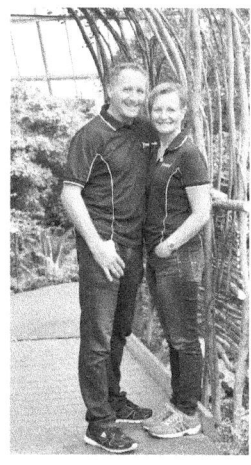

REFERENCES

Britannica, E. (n.d.). *Simon Magus.* Retrieved from https://www.brittanica.com/biography/Simon-Magus.

Bynum, W. (1994). *Science and the Practice of Medicine in the Nineteenth Century.* Cambridge University Press.

Cook, H. J. (2011). The History of Medicine and the Scientific Revolution. *Isis, vol 102 (1)*, 102–108.

Crutchfield, L. (1991). *The Origins of Dispensationalism: The Darby Factor.* University Press of America.

Dossey, B. (2000). *Florence Nightingale: Mystic, Visionary, Healer.* Springhouse Corporation.

Finocchiaro, M. (1989). *The Galileo Affair: A Documentary History.* University of California Press.

Gatti, H. (1999). *Giordono Bruno and Renaissance Science: Broken Lives and Organizational Power.* Cornell University Press.

Harris, R. (2000). *Lourdes: Body and Spirit in the Secular Age.* Penguin Books.

Judd, D. A. (2013). *The History of Nursing.* Jones and Bartlett Learning.

Koenig, H. G. (2000). Religion and Medicine 1: Historical Background and Reasons for Separation. *International Journal of Psychiatry in Medicine, 30(4)*, 385–398.

Miller, T. (1997). *The Birth of the Hospital in the Byzantine Empire.* John Hopkins University Press.

Myrick, C. S. (2009). The Separation of Church and Medicine. *AMA Journal of Ethics, 11(10)*, 747–749.

Pattison, S. (2010). Religion and the Secularization of Health Care. *Journal of Clinical Nursing, 19(17-18)*, 2327–2335.

Porter, R. (1997). *The Greatest Benefit of Mankind: A Medical History of Humanity from Antiquity to the Present.* HarperCollins.

Post, S. G. (2009). The Separation of Church and Medicine. *AMA Journal of Ethics, 11(10)*, 744–747.

Rosen, E. (1995). *Copernicus and His Successors.* The Hambledon Press.

Rosenberg, E. C. (1987). *The Care of Strangers: The Rise of America's Hospital System.* John Hopkins University Press.

Sweetnam, M. M. (2009). *The Scofield Bible: Its History and Impact on the Evangelical Church.* Authentic USA.

NOTES

1. River of Life

1. "Spring Up, O Well, Spring Up," written by Mary A. Lathbury, 1895, public domain.

3. Trouble with Theology

1. (Sweetnam, 2009), (Crutchfield, 1991).

6. Education Is Good

1. Spencer Johnson, MD, *Who Moved My Cheese?: An A-Mazing Way to Deal with Change in Your Work and in Your Life* (New York: Putnam, 1998).
2. (Finocchiaro, 1989).
3. (Gatti, 1999).
4. (Rosen, 1995).

7. What Is Good Health?

1. World Health Organization, "Constitution of the World Health Organization," 1946, https://www.who.int/about/governance/constitution.
2. World Health Organization, "Health Promotion," https://www.who.int/health-topics/health-promotion#tab=tab_1.
3. Global CHE Network, "What Is Good Health?" in *Community Health Evangelism* curriculum.

10. The Medical Priesthood

1. (Britannica, n.d.).
2. (Miller, 1997), (Rosenberg, 1987).
3. (Porter, 1997).
4. (Judd, 2013).
5. (Dossey, 2000).
6. (Post, 2009).
7. (Koenig, 2000).
8. (Bynum, 1994), (Myrick, 2009).
9. (Pattison, 2010).
10. (Cook, 2011).
11. (Harris, 2000).
12. Gwen Bergquist, *Destiny by Design*, https://destinybydesign.org.

ABOUT THE AUTHOR

Rhonda Hamilton is an Advanced Practice Registered Nurse with a career spanning nearly four decades in nursing. A true nurse's nurse, she is passionate about whole-person care, addressing the physical, emotional, and spiritual needs of her patients. Rhonda has dedicated much of her career to community health, both nationally and internationally, bringing compassionate care to some of the world's most vulnerable populations.

Her commitment to nursing excellence has been recognized through awards for direct patient care and community health, but her greatest reward is witnessing lives transformed through acts of mercy. Rhonda firmly believes that healing extends beyond medicine and into the realm of faith—where physical, emotional, and spiritual restoration intersect.

Rhonda's life's purpose is clear: to see people healed, whole, and empowered to walk in the fullness of health that God intends for them. In *Flow: Releasing a River of Healing into Healthcare*, Rhonda shares her journey of faith, doubt, and ultimately stepping into the calling of healing alongside God, challenging fellow healthcare professionals to do the same.

Beyond her professional work, Rhonda is a devoted wife, married to her husband, Rick, for more than thirty-five years. She is also a loving mother and grandmother, finding joy in family and faith.

www.ingramcontent.com/pod-product-compliance
Lightning Source LLC
Chambersburg PA
CBHW070923130626
46555CB00001B/252